Animal Physiologic Surgery

Contributors

EDWIN J. ANDREWS, Department of Veterinary Pathology, New York State College of Veterinary Medicine, Cornell University, Ithaca, NY

HOWARD C. HUGHES, V.M.D., Department of Comparative Medicine, The Milton S. Hershey Medical Center of The Pennsylvania State University, Hershey, PA

C. MAX LANG, Department of Comparative Medicine, The Milton S. Hershey Medical Center of The Pennsylvania State University, Hershey, PA

CAROLE A. MANCUSO, Department of Comparative Medicine, The Milton S. Hershey Medical Center of The Pennsylvania State University, Hershey, PA

WILLIAM J. WHITE, Department of Comparative Medicine, The Milton S. Hershey Medical Center of The Pennsylvania State University, Hershey, PA

ANIMAL PHYSIOLOGIC SURGERY

C. Max Lang

with 54 illustrations

Springer-Verlag

NEW YORK   HEIDELBERG   BERLIN

1976

EDWIN J. ANDREWS, V.M.D., Ph.D., Associate Professor,
Department of Veterinary Pathology,
New York State College of Veterinary Medicine,
Cornell University,
Ithaca, NY

HOWARD C. HUGHES, V.M.D., Professor,
Department of Comparative Medicine,
The Milton S. Hershey Medical Center of
The Pennsylvania State University,
Hershey, PA

C. MAX LANG, D.V.M., Professor and Chairman,
Department of Comparative Medicine,
The Milton S. Hershey Medical Center of
The Pennsylvania State University,
Hershey, PA

CAROLE A. MANCUSO, R.N., B.S.N.,
Department of Comparative Medicine,
The Milton S. Hershey Medical Center of
The Pennsylvania State University,
Hershey, PA

WILLIAM J. WHITE, V.M.D., Assistant Professor,
Department of Comparative Medicine,
The Milton S. Hershey Medical Center of
The Pennsylvania State University,
Hershey, PA

Library of Congress Cataloging in Publication Data

Lang, Max C.
   Animal physiologic surgery.

   Bibliography: p. 175
   Includes index.
   1. Veterinary physiology. 2. Veterinary surgery. I. Lang, Carol Max.
SF768.A48   636.089'2   76–15020

© 1976 by Springer-Verlag New York

Printed in the United States of America

ISBN 0-387-90187-6   Springer-Verlag   New York

ISBN 0-540-90187-6   Springer-Verlag   Berlin   Heidelberg

dedicated to Dr. George T. Harrell, in recognition of his contributions to medical education.

Preface

Animal Physiologic Surgery presents an integrated approach to the study of surgery for first-year medical students and graduate students in physiology. The primary emphasis is on the interrelationships between surgical techniques and physiologic phenomena observed before, during, and after surgery.

All procedures described in the book are designed so that the student with a limited knowledge of surgery can successfully assume responsibility for pre- and postoperative care, as well as for the operation. Therefore, the attitude reflected in this work shows the student his obligation, and his privilege, to find the best method of treatment for the patient and to work at his highest capacity.

The text begins with an introduction to operating-room procedures, sutures and instruments, wound healing, anesthesia, and water and electrolyte balance. The second part deals with step-by-step surgical instructions and clinical consideration in techniques, such as laparotomy, splenectomy, nephrectomy, and laminectomy. This part is followed by a section on laboratory techniques necessary for following and evaluating the course of the patient and on postmortem techniques.

The text strikes a balance between exacting detail and discussion of basic principles; it is easily adaptable to any curriculum.

I am grateful to the contributors for their close cooperation, especially Dr. William J. White for sharing much of the responsibilities. I am also very appreciative to Catherine Jackson and Anne Kupstas for their valuable editorial assistance, and to Joyce Greene and Becky Robertson for their assistance in preparing the manuscript.

I am indebted to Dr. George T. Harrell for his support and encouragement in developing the course that resulted in this text. The underlying philosophy of a strong educational base and the requirement for excellent patient care are directly attributable to his teachings.

C. Max Lang

Contents

II

Surgical Procedures

III

Laboratory Techniques

I

Introduction to Surgery

Although successful surgery requires a thorough knowledge of anatomy and physiology and a certain degree of manual dexterity, it also requires that the surgeon understand the principles of wound healing and of maintaining homeostasis. A suitable environment is also important to the success of an operation. In Chapters 1 through 5 some of the fundamentals of surgery are discussed.

1

Operating-Room Procedures

C. MAX LANG AND CAROLE A. MANCUSO

I. Introduction

The operating room is a specialized treatment area that must be run according to proven principles, whether the patients are animals or human beings. In order to fulfill his responsibility to his animal patients, the student must familiarize himself with all available resources and equipment of the area and their purpose or function. These include the following items:

Areas
    Reference library
    Dressing room
    Storage room for supplies
    Anesthesia and prep room
    Scrub room
    Operating room(s)
    Recovery room
    Laboratories
    Postmortem room
Equipment
    Surgical lights and table
    Instrument tray
    Sutures and needles
    Dressings and sponges
    Intravenous (i.v.) setup

Suction apparatus
Anesthesia machine
Cardiac cart
Resuscitators
Procedures and techniques
Principles of sterilization
Skin preparation and draping of the patient
Positioning of the patient
Scrub routine
Gowning and gloving routine
Conductivity testing
Duties of surgical team members
Sponge counting
Blood and specimen collection
Postoperative care
Necropsy techniques

In addition to being familiar with all of the equipment and techniques listed above, each person participating in an operation must have a complete understanding of the basic aims of the procedure and of his or her role. The importance of developing good habits, cooperative teamwork, and self-discipline cannot be overstressed. The following principles should be instilled into each student:

1. Treatment of the patient is the sole purpose of the operating room, and all activity must be directed to his care.
2. Any general surgical procedure is an intrusive alteration to a patient's physiology and anatomy and should be considered as an event of major importance in his life.
3. To serve the needs of all—patients and surgeons—a scheduled routine must be maintained.
4. Safety for the patient, other team members, and yourself is of prime consideration.
5. Routines such as gowning, gloving, suturing, etc., require practice before they are used in the operating room.
6. Strict asepsis is an absolute necessity. If there is any doubt as to whether sterile technique has been broken, one should correct the contaminated condition at once.
7. Gentleness in dealing with the patient and in handling the tissues will promote healing.
8. Surgical instruments are usually quite delicate and are made for a specific purpose.

9. The surgical equipment and supplies are expensive and should be used carefully and economically.
10. If you are unsure about any aspect of an operation, ask someone and make sure that you completely understand before proceeding.

II. Sterilization

While basic principles of aseptic technique are important in all aspects of medicine, strict adherence to these principles is mandatory in the operating room. Therefore, each surgical suite has established regulations which apply to that particular environment; although the actual procedures may vary from place to place, the basic principles remain the same.

Ideally, the maintenance of asepsis means the elimination of all pathogenic organisms from the operating room. Although this ideal cannot always be attained, every effort should be made to approach it by strictly observing the following measures:

1. Sterilization of everything possible in the environment of a surgical procedure.
2. Decontamination of the patient by general cleanliness and meticulous preparation of the incision site.
3. Adherence to established rules concerning attire, conduct, and routines by all operating-room personnel.
4. Environmental control of pathogens by:
   a. Adequate and scientific control of air pressure and exchanges in the room.
   b. Strict housekeeping and clean-up procedures.
   c. Restriction of traffic through the area.
   d. Complete cooperation of all who do enter the surgical areas.

The effectiveness of this program should be monitored routinely by means of bacteriologic cultures. Evaluation af all aspects of operative techniques and wound healing is also essential to assure the adequacy of the sanitation program.

Sterilization of instruments, clothing, and equipment can be done in several different ways. The following methods are used:

1. Saturated steam under pressure, usually in an autoclave. The temperature, pressure, and time must be adjusted according to the type of material and the size of the load to be sterilized. The

recommended standards are as shown in the following tabulation.

Temperature (°F)	Pressure (lb)	Minimum time (min)
250	15	15
262	20	5
270	27–30	3

Special attention must be given to wrapping articles and loading the autoclave to make sure that there is sufficient space for steam penetration and subsequent drying of the load. The high-vacuum autoclaves have the advantage of completing the process in a shorter period of time.

2. Chemical sterilization. Gas sterilization with ethylene oxide is an effective method for those materials and/or pieces of equipment that would be damaged by heat. Articles sterilized by this process must be aerated for one week after sterilization to eliminate any invisible chemical residue that may be harmful if absorbed into the body. The most effective chemical solution for sterilizing articles that may be damaged by steam is a commercial glutaraldehyde product. However, it is essential to adhere strictly to the manufacturer's recommendation to avoid damage to the article.

3. Dry-heat sterilization. This method of sterilization is done in special hot-air ovens at 320°F.

4. Electronic beam (DNA ionizing radiation). This form of sterilization is most commonly used in industry for prepackaged materials.

Several other procedures that are often used for sterilization are not routinely effective. Boiling water is not considered to be an adequate means of sterilization because it does not destroy spores. Boiling for 20 minutes or longer, however, will destroy the vegetative forms of organisms. Many liquid chemicals used for decontamination will not ensure complete sterility. The chemicals commonly used for decontamination are individually classified as antiseptics, germicides, or bactericides, and they must be used accordingly. Machines producing ultrasonic waves are used for cleaning instruments but are not a means of sterilization.

III. Operative Procedure

In this course the operative procedure is defined as beginning when the patient enters the surgical area and ending when the patient reaches the recovery room, the surgical record is completed, and the operating room areas are cleaned. The basic steps, in sequential fashion, are as follows:

1. Anesthetize the patient, insert the endotracheal tube, and insert a needle for i.v. injections.
2. Carry out preliminary preparation of the incision area by shaving the hair and cleansing the skin.
3. Position and secure the patient on the operating table.
4. Scrub hands, put on gown, and then gloves.
5. Prepare the instrument table and suture materials.
6. Finish preparing the patient's skin, applying an antiseptic to the incision line first, then working outward until the entire operative area, or six inches around the proposed incision site, is covered. A clean sponge should be used if additional antiseptic is applied to the incision site.
7. Drape the patient.
8. Make the incision.
9. Explore the operative area, using sponges or towels wet with normal saline (a 0.9% solution of sodium chloride) to pack off the viscera.
10. Carry out the operative procedure.
11. Count sponges and instruments according to individual operating room procedure.
12. Close the incision.
13. Recount sponges and instruments.
14. Clean and dress the wound, using a sterile, dry sponge or Vaseline gauze on the incision line and sterile sponges wet with saline for the outer areas; secure the dressing with adhesive. An alternative method is to use a colloidal type of spray.
15. Place the patient in a comfortable position in the recovery room. Remove the water bowl and any objects with which the patient could injure himself while recovering from the anesthesia.
16. Record the operative procedure, using the correct title of the operation and an exact description of the anatomy and of the techniques used.
17. Remain with patient until the endotracheal tube can be removed and the patient is conscious enough to right himself.

18. Clean the operating room, discarding all disposable needles, syringes, and knife blades in a specific disposal box.

A. Operating-room attire

Personal hygiene and cleanliness on the part of all personnel are necessary for maintaining aseptic technique. No one should enter the operating suite who has not bathed thoroughly that day and whose fingernails are not clipped short. Anyone participating in the operation should remove all watches, bracelets, and rings, along with all street clothing (shirt, pants, dresses, and any underclothing

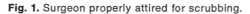

Fig. 1. Surgeon properly attired for scrubbing.

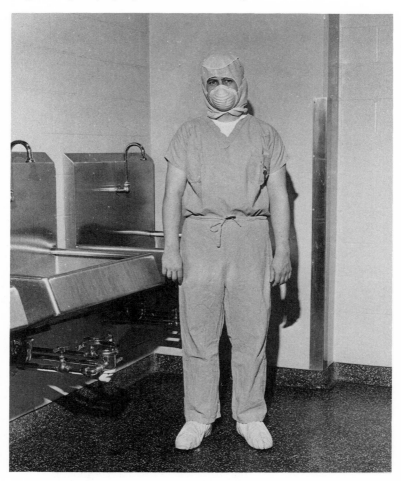

or hosiery that may cause static electricity). These items are locked in a dressing-room locker, and the key is pinned to the scrub suit or dress. The operating-room attire is provided for a specific operating room and should be worn only in that suite. Scrub shirts must be tucked into the pants (Fig. 1). Sleeves should be rolled to 3 inches above the elbows, and trouser legs should end at the ankles. The scrub dresses should be belted comfortably. Scrub clothing is more comfortable if it is too large than if it is too small. The scalp hair should be completely covered by a scrub cap or a special hood mask (Fig. 2) designed to cover long scalp and facial hair.

Fig. 2. Surgeon wearing surgical hood.

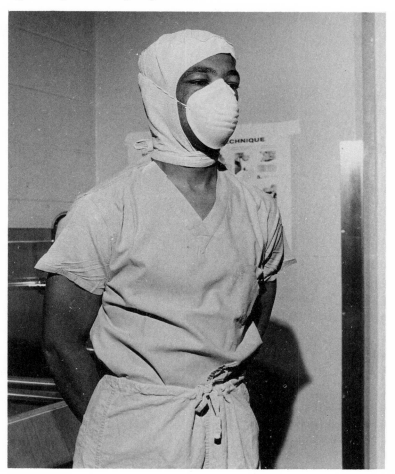

Face masks must be worn at all times in the operating room. After the hands have been washed, the mask is placed comfortably over the face in such a manner that subsequent adjustment will not be necessary. If eyeglasses are worn, the top of the mask should be adjusted to prevent fogging. The mask should be removed at the end of the operation and should never be worn dangling about the neck or up on the head.

Even though shoe covers are provided, shoes must be clean and preferably reserved for use in the operating room. Just before

Fig. 3. The conductivity of the shoe covers is tested by standing on a conductivity tester.

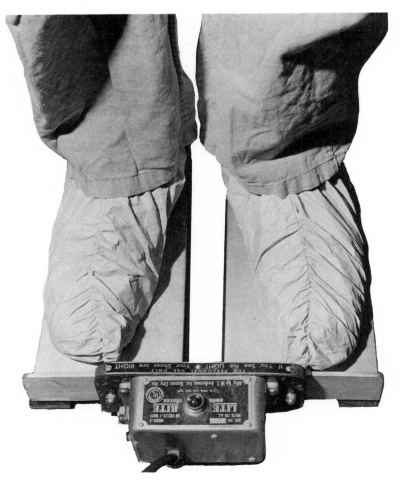

scrubbing, the shoe covers should be put on. There are many types of conductive shoe covers that can be worn in the operating room, and it is important to follow the recommendations of the manufacturer and to test the conductivity of the shoe covers after they are on the feet (Fig. 3).

B. Surgical scrub routine

There are several modifications of the surgical scrub routine, most of which are effective. The following method is a simplified procedure which, if done correctly, meets the basic criteria for aseptic surgery.

1. Thoroughly wet the hands and arms under running water to approximately 2 inches above the elbows. Avoid wetting the outer clothing.
2. To prevent recontamination of the hands, hold them high, with the elbows flexed and away from the body, at all times.
3. Apply liquid soap solution to the hands (Fig. 4A) and work up a good lather.
4. Wash the hands and arms thoroughly to 2 inches above the elbows for at least one minute or until they are visibly clean. Clean under and around the fingernails with a sterile orange-wood stick (Fig. 4B), which is then discarded.
5. Rinse well from the fingertips to the elbows.
6. Take a sterile brush or sponge from the dispenser and add liquid soap (unless it is presoaped). Brush the fingernails of each hand for 50 strokes.
7. Rinse thoroughly from the fingertips to the elbows.
8. Using the sterile brush or sponge, scrub for 5 minutes or 20 circular strokes to each skin area of the hands, wrist, and arms, in that order (Fig. 4C). If adequate suds are not made by adding small amounts of water to the brush, rinse well and repeat the scrub in the same order.
9. Touching the fingers lightly together, rinse thoroughly from the fingertips to the elbows (Fig. 4D) and allow the excess water to drain from the arms before leaving the sink.

C. Gowning routine

Although the gowns are sterile when they are unwrapped, the surgeon should consider the gown as sterile only in the area from the midchest to the draped table level; the sleeves can be considered sterile from the wrists to the elbows. The following procedure is recommended:

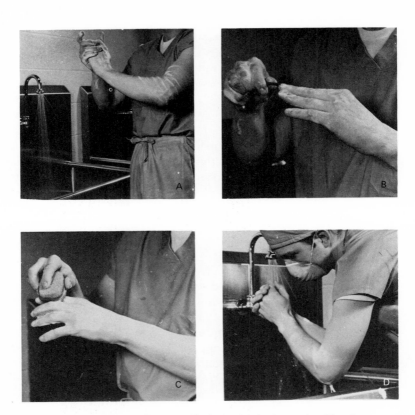

Fig. 4. Surgical scrub. After a preliminary 1-minute wash without a brush (A), the fingernails are cleaned with a sterile orange-wood stick (B). The fingers and hands are scrubbed (at least 50 strokes) with a sterile brush (C), then rinsed under running water (D).

1. Have the circulating nurse open the outer wrap of the sterile towel and gown.
2. Grasp the towel fold with one hand and *lift* the towel away from the wrapper (Fig. 5A); do not drag it off.
3. With the arms held away from the body, dry the hands well, using a different area of the towel for each hand. Drying should be done by firm strokes. Dry each arm with one upward spiral movement of the towel from the wrist to the elbow (Fig. 5B). Do not allow the towel to touch the scrub suit.
4. Discard the towel in a bucket or on an unsterile table.
5. Grasp the gown at the fold, lift it up, and back away from the table (Fig. 6A).

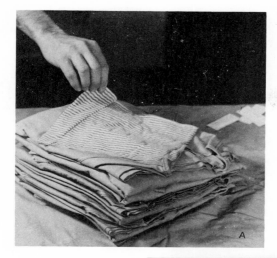

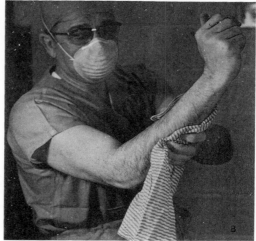

Fig. 5. Drying the hands and arms. (A) The sterile towel is removed from the pack. (B) After both hands have been patted dry the arm is dried in one spiral motion.

6. Hold the shoulder fold of the gown in the other hand, thus, allowing it to open (Fig. 6B). It must be held high enough so that it does not touch anything.
7. Do not touch any other part of the gown's exterior surface.
8. Look for the sleeve seams and gently slip first one hand and then the other into the openings (Fig. 6C). Do not attempt to

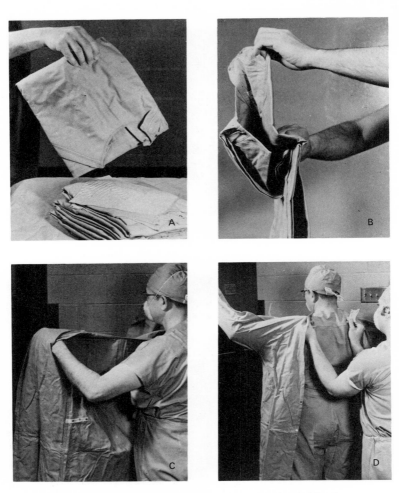

Fig. 6. Gowning. After removing the gown from the pack (A), the surgeon opens the gown (B) and inserts his arms into the armholes (C). The circulating nurse then fastens the back grippers (D).

push the hands through the wrist openings. The circulating nurse will pull the sleeves up and fasten the back grippers (Fig. 6D). Those wearing wrap-around gowns should have the side grippers fastened by a sterile-gloved assistant rather than the circulating nurse.

D. Gloving routine

Surgical gloves are usually prepowdered. The surgeon should choose a size that will allow for some slight swelling without discomfort. Either the closed or the open gloving routine can be used.

1. Closed Gloving Routine:
   a. After putting on the gown, do not push the hands through the gown wristlets.
   b. Grasp the left glove with the left hand through the material of the gown sleeve, being very careful not to touch the unsterile edge of the glove wrap.
   c. Rest the folded glove on the left sleeve with the palm against the gown sleeve and with the fingers pointing toward the elbow, while grasping the cuff tightly through the gown material (Fig. 7A).
   d. With the gown-covered right hand, pull the left glove cuff completely over the gown wristlet (Fig. 7B).
   e. Repeat this process for the right hand, using the gloved left hand (Fig. 7C).
   f. The circulating nurse will then pull the sleeves up and fasten the back grippers of the gown.
2. Open Gloving Routine:
   a. Push the hands through the gown wristlets as the circulating nurse pulls the sleeves up.
   b. Left glove. With the right hand, grasp the folded-over surface (the surface that will be next to the skin) on the palm side of the cuff and lift the glove away from the wrapper (Fig. 8A). Use a gentle, side-to-side motion to draw the glove over the hand (Fig. 8B), being careful not to touch the gown with your bare hand; leave the cuff turned down.
   c. Right glove. With the right hand, grasp the cuff on the folded-over surface; lift the glove away from the wrap and place the gloved left hand under the cuff, touching only the sterile side (Fig. 8C). Draw the glove over the right hand and bring the cuff up over the gown wristlet.
   d. Place the gloved right fingers under the left cuff and pull it up over the gown wristlet.

After gloving, the surgeon should always keep his hands above the waist and next to the sterile area of the gown.

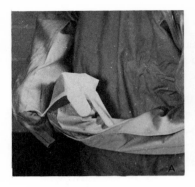
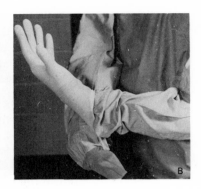

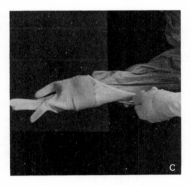

Fig. 7. Closed gloving technique. (A) To pull the left glove over the gown wristlet, both sides of the cuff are grasped with gown-covered fingers. (B) With the gown-covered right hand, the left glove is pulled on. (C) The gloved left hand touches only the sterile side of the right glove as it pulls it on.

E. Removal of operating-room attire

To protect personnel from contamination by any bacteria that may be on the used gown and gloves, the surgeon should remove the gloves, gown, and mask as carefully as he put them on. The following procedure is recommended:

1. While still at the operating table, use a clean wet towel to wipe off the gloves (Fig. 9A); discard the towel in the hamper.
2. Have the circulating nurse open the gown grippers.
3. Remove the gown by drawing it (soiled side down) away from the body over the gloves (Fig. 9B).

16

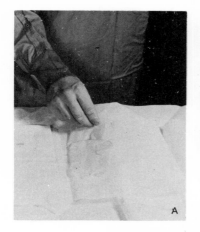
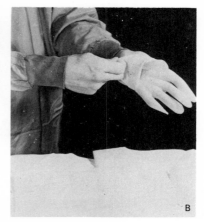
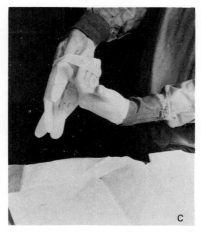

Fig. 8. Open gloving technique. The left glove is removed from
the pack (A) and held by the fold of the cuff as it is pulled over
the hand (B). The gloved left hand touches only the sterile side
of the right glove as it pulls it on (C).

4. Fold the soiled side in and discard the garment in the hamper.
5. Place the soiled side of one glove under the other glove cuff to
   remove it (Fig. 9C).
6. Place the ungloved hand under the skin side of the remaining
   glove cuff and remove it (Fig. 9D).
7. Wash hands and arms thoroughly with soap and water.
8. Grasp the ties of the mask; remove and discard it carefully. Do
   not touch the outer surface of the mask with your hands.

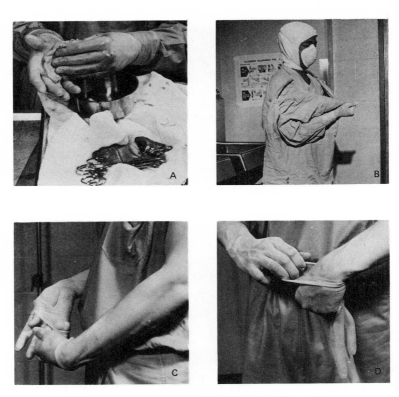

Fig. 9. Degowning. After wiping the gloved hands with a wet towel at the operating table (A), the surgeon removes first the gown (B), then the right glove (C), and then the left (D).

IV. General Conduct

Conversation should be kept to a minimum and restricted to the operative procedure. A quiet environment affords less distraction and less chance for error.

Any surgical procedure requires team effort, and the responsibilities of each member of the team should be clearly defined by the surgeon before the operation begins. Some of these responsibilities are preparing and draping the patient, maintaining the best possible illumination of the operative field at all times, providing exposure of the operative area by proper positioning of the patient and the gentle but effective use of retractors, continual "housekeeping" to prevent the accumulation of instruments, sponges, and pieces of suture material, keeping the field free of blood and the tissues moist. The entire team must constantly be alert to avoid a break in sterile technique.

Scalpels and needles are very sharp instruments by which the surgeon or his assistants may be injured. The scalpel is designed to make an incision and should be held only when in use; at other times, it belongs on the instrument tray. It is not uncommon for someone to be stuck accidentally by a needle. All injuries should immediately be brought to the attention of the instructor.

Although the surgeon is specifically charged with seeing the animal safely through the operation, both the surgeon and the assistant are intimately concerned with the technical aspects of the procedure and both should have a complete understanding of the anatomy of the area and its physiologic functions.

The assistant should be able to substitute for the surgeon if necessary. Usually, however, his work complements that of the surgeon. He exposes, sponges, places forceps, removes hemostats, etc. Complete cooperation between the surgeon and his assistant helps to ensure an efficient and successful operation.

2

Instruments and Sutures

C. MAX LANG AND CAROLE A. MANCUSO

I. Instruments (Figs. 10–12)

Surgical instruments are expensive, and each instrument is manufactured precisely and scientifically for a specific function. The student surgeon should learn the specific function of each instrument and to do any procedure with the very basic instruments, so that he can acquire efficiency and dexterity in their use. For clarity of communication with other members of the surgical team, it is important for the student surgeon to learn the correct name for each instrument, as well as its proper use.

The basic surgery pack usually includes the following instruments:

    1. Cutting instruments (Fig. 10)
       A. Scalpel
       B. Scissors
          (1) Bandage scissors
          (2) Iris scissors
          (3) Mayo dissecting scissors
          (4) Metzenbaum scissors
          (5) Suture scissors
          (6) Wire scissors
       C. Grooved director
    2. Crushing and grasping instruments (Fig. 11)
       A. Allis tissue forceps

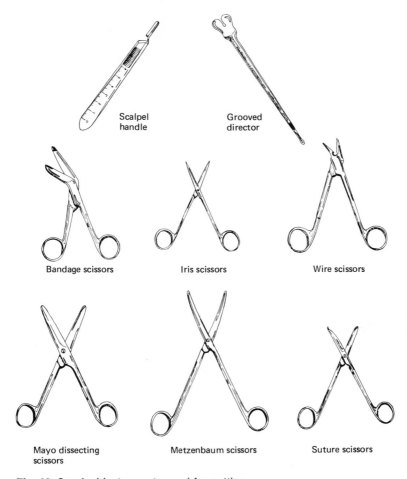

Fig. 10. Surgical instruments used for cutting.

    B. Dressing and tissue forceps
    C. Hemostatic forceps
       (1) Halstead mosquito forceps
       (2) Kelly forceps
       (3) Mixter forceps
    D. Sponge-holding forceps
    E. Backhaus towel clamp
    F. Needle-holder
  3. Retractors (Fig. 12)
    A. Balfour abdominal retractor

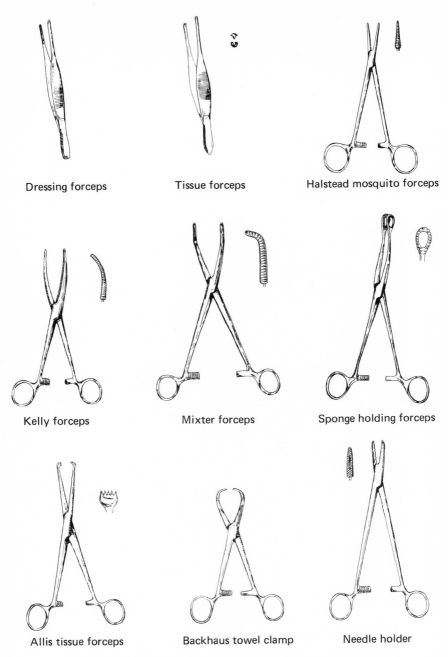

Dressing forceps

Tissue forceps

Halstead mosquito forceps

Kelly forceps

Mixter forceps

Sponge holding forceps

Allis tissue forceps

Backhaus towel clamp

Needle holder

Fig. 11. Surgical instruments used for crushing and grasping.

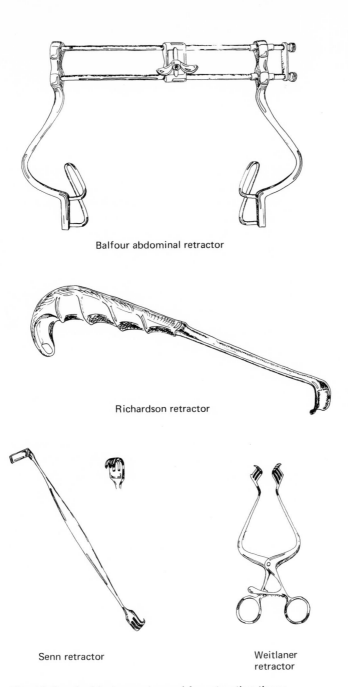

Balfour abdominal retractor

Richardson retractor

Senn retractor

Weitlaner
retractor

Fig. 12. Surgical instruments used for retracting tissue.

B. Richardson retractor
C. Senn retractor
D. Weitlaner retractor

II. Sutures

A. Suture materials

A suture is a cord, thread, or wire that is used to sew tissues together. A ligature is a cord or thread used to tie off blood vessels. Common usage, however, has established *suture* as a generic term for all materials used as sutures or ligatures.

Sutures are classified as being either absorbable or nonabsorbable. Suture materials that are absorbed by the body over a period of days or weeks include surgical gut and fascia lata. Nonabsorbable sutures (which remain in place unless removed) are made of materials such as silk, linen, cotton, wire, and various synthetics. A good suture material has the following characteristics:

1. It is capable of being sterilized.
2. It is free of irritating substances.
3. It is pliable enough to tie.
4. It holds the knot securely, at least until healing has occurred.
5. It has a fine gauge.
6. It has sufficient tensile strength to hold the edges of the wound in apposition.
7. It will support the tissues until healing has occurred.
8. When it has served its function, it will be absorbed by the body or can remain without causing a foreign-body reaction.

Of the absorbable suture materials, surgical gut, or catgut, is the one most commonly used. *Catgut* is actually a misnomer, since this suture material is made from the small intestine of young sheep. The submucosa, after being freed from the rest of the intestinal wall by treatment with chemicals and enzymes, is washed and cut into strips. These are then twisted into strings containing varying numbers of strips, or plies. The more strips, the larger is the diameter of the resultant strand and the greater its tensile strength.

Surgical gut is supplied in two forms: plain and chromic. The former, because it has not been chemically treated, is more rapidly absorbed by the tissues. The latter is treated with chromium salts to delay absorption. There are four standard types of surgical gut, classified according to absorbability (see tabulation on next page).

Although surgical gut comes in sizes ranging from 0000000

Type	Treatment	Duration of tensile strength in tissues (days)
A	None	3–7
B	Mild chromic	7–10
C	Medium chromic	12–15
D	Extra chromic	20–25

(seven aught) to 7, the size most commonly used is 00, which has a diameter between 0.0254 and 0.0330 cm. The minimum tensile strength required for unknotted 00 surgical gut on a straight pull is 5 pounds. The effective tensile strength in a strand of surgical gut is reduced when a knot is tied in it, because of fraying of the strand.

B. Knot tying

Dexterity and speed in tying knots can be acquired only by practice—and the student should practice tying knots until it becomes automatic, requiring no concentration at all. The knot must be tied firmly, so that it will not slip; but the tissues must not be drawn together so tightly as to impede healing. Although a wide variety of complicated knots can be used, the student surgeon should concentrate on the square knot.

The student should learn to tie knots with a needle holder, as well as with his fingers. He will find the needle holder method useful when the end of the suture is short or when his suture material or gloves are slippery. The standard method is to grasp the short end of the suture with a needle holder, about which has been looped the long end, and pull snugly. If this maneuver is repeated twice, a triple knot results; if a second knot is tied as a mirror image of the first, the result is a square knot (Fig. 13). The needle holder should be applied only to the ends of sutures, because the sharp jaws of this instrument will tend to break the fibers it holds.

C. Suture needles (Fig. 14)

Suture needles come in many varieties and sizes and may be either straight or curved. Curved needles are used primarily when it is difficult or impossible to bring to the surface of the wound the tissues being sewed together.

The points of suture needles may be tapered (round) or may have a cutting edge like a bayonet, spear, or trocar. Except where

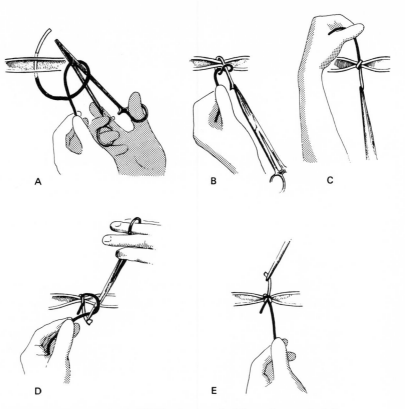

Fig. 13. The square knot. (A) The long end of the suture material (black) grasped firmly in the left hand is looped over the hemostat held in the right hand. (B) The free end of the suture material (white) is grasped with the hemostat and pulled through the loop toward the surgeon. (C) The long strand is then pulled away from the surgeon while the other end is pulled toward the surgeon, thus, tightening the first throw of the knot. (D) The jaws of the hemostat are opened, releasing the suture material, while the long end of the suture material (still held firmly in the left hand) is looped over the hemostat. The hemostat is then used to grasp the short end of the suture material. (E) The short end of the suture material is pulled through the loop away from the surgeon while the long end is pulled toward him, completing the knot.

tissue resistance (in the skin, for example) demands a cutting point for easy penetration, tapered needles should be used exclusively, since they produce a minimum of trauma. The elastic

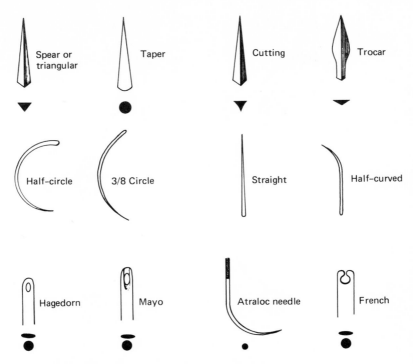

Fig. 14. Points, shafts, and eyes of surgical needles.

tissues soon obliterate the small, circular hole made by the round point; whereas the needles with a cutting edge leave a pathway through the tissue, so that undue tension on the suture may cause it to tear.

Needles may have eyes like ordinary sewing needles (Hagedorn, Mayo needles); they may be eyeless and swaged (attached to the end of the suture) or they may have spring eyes (French needle). Swaged, atraloc, needles (attached to the end of the suture) are normally used for delicate work where it is essential to minimize trauma.

Needles should be threaded carefully from the inside (if curved) without tension, which may cause fraying (Fig. 15). The needle may be threaded twice to keep the suture material from pulling out (Fig. 16). When delicate suturing is being done, it is better to thread the needle only once, in order to reduce the size of the knot. In this case, the surgeon must pull on the thread and not on the needle to make the suture taut.

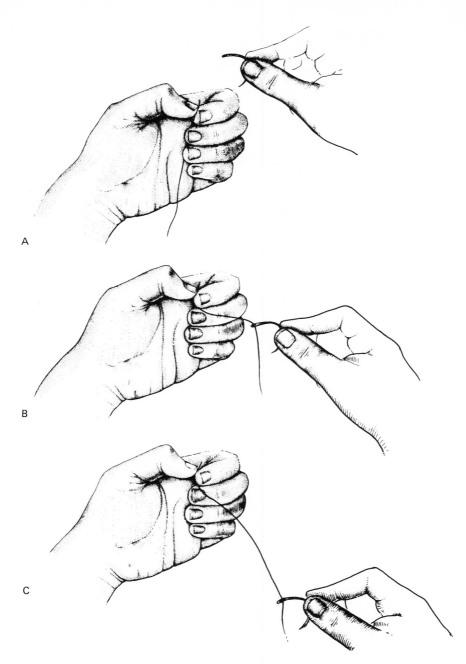

Fig. 15. Proper method of holding a curved needle and threading it from the inside.

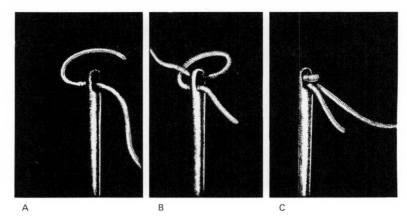

A   B   C

Fig. 16. Double-threading a needle.

III. Suturing (Figs. 17–19)

Good apposition of tissues is dependent on choosing the right suture material, needle, and pattern and then using them properly. A needle is less likely to break and is more easily directed if it is held along the shank rather than near the point or the eye. Trauma can be minimized by using the smallest needle that will do the job.

There are many varieties of suture patterns (Figs. 17, 18 and 19), but the beginning surgeon should attempt to master only the few basic patterns that are routinely used. The choice of pattern should be based on three criteria: (1) Will it hold the tissues in the required position without undue tension? (2) Does it distribute tension on the suture material and tissue in such a manner as not to exceed the tensile strength of the suture material? (3) Does it require a minimal amount of suture material?

A. Removal of sutures

Removal of exposed sutures should be done some time between the fourth and the fourteenth postoperative day, depending on (1) the extent of the wound, (2) evidence of infection, and (3) the physical stress to which the wound may be subjected.

If healing is by first intention and the scar is supported by underlying sutures or is in a location where movement is slight, the skin sutures may safely be removed as early as the fourth or fifth day postoperatively. If healing is delayed for any reason, the

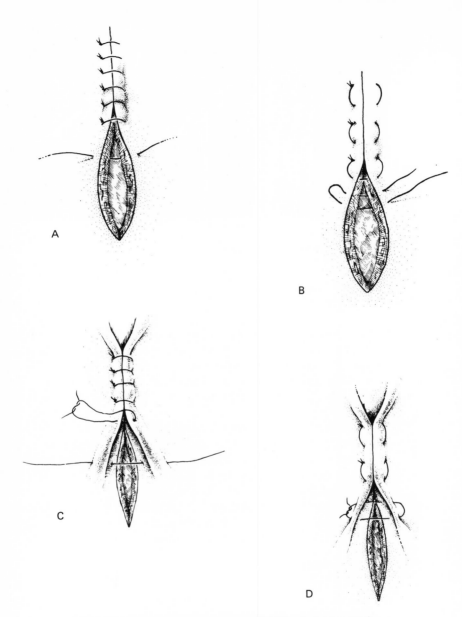

Fig. 17. Interrupted suture patterns. (A) Simple interrupted sutures. (B) Interrupted horizontal mattress sutures. (C) Interrupted vertical mattress sutures. (D) Halsted sutures (inverted horizontal mattress sutures).

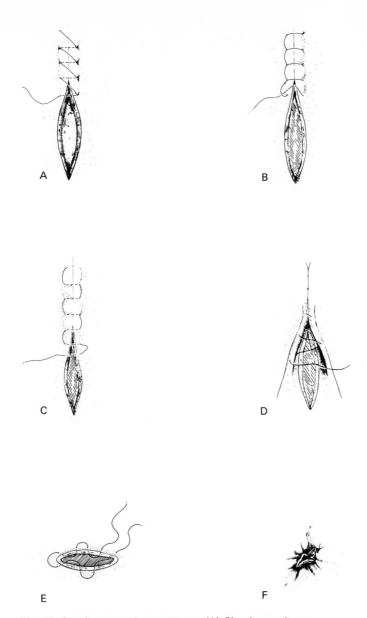

Fig. 18. Continuous suture patterns. (A) Simple continuous suture (through-and-through suture). (B) Simple continuous lock stitch. (C) Continuous horizontal mattress suture. (D) Continuous Lembert suture (continuous vertical mattress suture). (E) Purse-string suture, open and (F) closed.

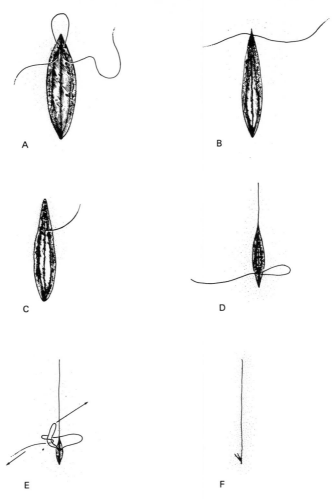

A   B

C   D

E   F

Fig. 19. Subcuticular closure with a continuous horizontal mattress suture. (A) The suture needle is inserted beneath the subcuticular tissue and brought out near the skin edge. The suture is then brought over the opposing skin edge and the needle is inserted through the subcuticular tissue and brought out beneath it. (B) As the knot is tied in a square knot, it buries itself beneath the subcuticular layer. (C) and (D) Sutures are placed 0.5 cm apart and should never penetrate the skin. It is advisable to include some of the underlying tissue in the suture pattern every 2 to 4 cm in order to eliminate "dead space" under the subcuticular layer. (E) The suture pattern is terminated by tying a buried knot, using a double strand of suture material and the end of the suture with the needle attached. (F) As the knot is tightened, it slips beneath the subcuticular layer.

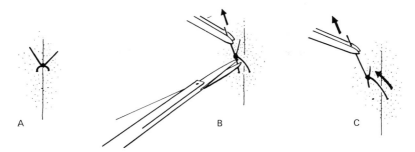

Fig. 20. Removal of a skin suture. (A) Surface of disinfected skin, showing skin suture. (B) One end of the suture is grasped with a pair of forceps and pulled upward at a right angle to the skin surface, thus exposing a portion of the suture that has been buried in the skin. The suture is cut at that point. (C) The suture is gently pulled out of the skin.

skin sutures should be left in longer. In long, weight-bearing incisions (such as midline abdominal incisions), the sutures should remain in place at least a week and sometimes as long as two weeks. It should be remembered, however, that scar tissue continues to form as long as the sutures remain in place.

In removing the sutures (Fig. 20), one must take care to avoid contamination of the wound. This will be less of a problem if the knots are tied to one side of the incision. After the incision and exposed portions of the sutures have been individually cleansed with an antiseptic, the sutures are removed by the method shown in Figure 20. When this method is used, only the clean portion of the suture is drawn through the tissues as it is pulled out. After all the sutures have been removed, the incision site should again be cleansed with an antiseptic.

3

Wound Healing

C. MAX LANG AND WILLIAM J. WHITE

The process of wound healing is basically the same, regardless of the kind of tissue involved, the type of injury, and the manner of its infliction (whether accidental or intentional). The primary difference between accidental and operative wounds lies in the fact that preparation for repair of the latter is made before the wound occurs.

Wound healing is arbitrarily divided into stages according to the activities of cell populations. Initially, blood flows into the opening created by the traumatic agent, fills the space and clots, thus, uniting the edges of the wound. During the next several hours this clot loses fluid; and the surface becomes dehydrated, forming a hard crust, or scab, which protects the wound as the healing process continues.

Inflammation of the wound begins as fluid from the adjacent blood vessels enter the wound. As a result of this swelling, additional pressure is placed on the suture line and the integrity of the suture knot. It is very important to allow space for this swelling, by not tying the sutures too tightly, when the wound is being sutured.

Approximately 6 hours after the injury, various types of white blood cells start to migrate into the wound and to attack and remove cellular debris as well as bacteria and foreign debris that may be present. Subsequently, fibroblasts enter the wound and manufacture collagen and other proteins to build scar tissue. As these fibroblasts synthesize collagen, large numbers of small blood vessels are formed throughout the wound. After the connective tissue structure of the wound has become reestablished, many of the capillaries regress.

The healing process can be delayed by many factors, including interference with blood supply to the wound, trauma by rough handling or improper use of instruments, foreign material, and improper closure. Any significant interference with the healing process can result in dehiscence, i.e., a disruption of the wound.

If it is necessary to reenter an incision site before the healing process is completed, the new incision must be made in the original site. If the reentry incision is lateral to the original site, this interruption in blood supply can cause necrosis of the tissue between the two incision lines. Before closing a healing wound, the surgeon should carefully debride the edges of each layer, i.e., excise the traumatized portion of the friable new material. This procedure will also help to ensure the correct identification and apposition of individual tissue layers.

It is the aim of surgery to bring about healing without complications. This can occur only when surgical trauma is kept to a minimum, strict asepsis is observed, and the divided tissues are carefully reunited.

4

Anesthesia

C. MAX LANG AND HOWARD C. HUGHES

The purpose of administering an anesthetic is to make the patient insensible to pain and incapable of movement. In general, animals are anesthetized by the same drugs and methods that are used for man. All laboratory animals should be anesthetized before being subjected to any surgical procedure. This chapter deals only with anesthesia in dogs, since the procedures described in this book are most commonly done in dogs.

I. Preanesthetic Medications

All supplies and equipment should be prepared in advance. Preanesthetic medications are often given to prevent apprehension, inhibit salivation, produce analgesia, and reduce the amount of anesthetic agent necessary to bring the animal to a surgical plane of anesthesia. The combination of preanesthetic medications employed most frequently in dogs consists of atropine (0.04 to 0.08 mg/kg given subcutaneously) together with morphine sulfate (4 mg/kg) or meperidine hydrochloride, U.S.P. (2 to 10 mg/kg subcutaneously). Morphine and meperidine are narcotics and have an analgesic as well as a sedative effect. Atropine is a parasympatholytic drug that prevents the interaction of acetylcholine with the effector cells, particularly in the heart and salivary glands. In addition to minimizing the emetic effect of morphine, atropine inhibits salivation and nasopharyngeal secretion and abolishes the vagolytic effects of barbiturate anesthesia.

The preanesthetic medications should be given 30 to 40 minutes prior to the induction of anesthesia, and the dog should be exercised to allow defecation and vomiting while the medications are taking effect.

II. Intravenous Anesthesia

Barbiturates given by i.v. injection are the anesthetic agents most commonly employed for dogs. The major action of the barbiturates is to depress the central nervous system and induce sleep.

Barbiturates offer the advantages of low cost and ease of administration, however, the anesthesia is less readily controlled as compared to inhalation anesthetics. Drugs injected into the bloodstream cease to act only after they are metabolized by the liver or excreted by the kidneys; whereas inhalation anesthetics are rapidly eliminated from the body. Another disadvantage of barbiturates is that the complete muscular relaxation required for some surgical procedures cannot be achieved with a dose that is entirely safe.

A. Injection into the cephalic vein

If an i.v. anesthetic is to be used, the dog's hair should be clipped over *both* cephalic veins. While other veins are sometimes used for the injection, the right cephalic is the most convenient if the assistant is right-handed. Clipping over both cephalic veins ensures that a secondary site for injection will be immediately available in case entry cannot be made into the primary site.

The injection of an intravenous agent requires two people: one to restrain the dog and one to make the injection. Both the anesthetist and his assistant should approach the dog in a friendly manner in order to allay anxiety. A right-handed assistant stands on the left side of the dog (Fig. 21) with his right hand around the dog's right foreleg. The ring and little fingers are curled behind the olecranon to prevent the dog from pulling his leg back (the index and middle fingers under the olecranon), and the thumb is placed on top of the leg to apply pressure to the cephalic vein and rotate it slightly laterally.

A syringe (usually 10 ml) is filled with the calculated amount of anesthetic solution, plus an extra 10% to allow for individual variation in dosage requirements. A 20- or 22-gauge, 1¼ inch needle is attached so that the bevel is facing in the same direction as the syringe calibration.

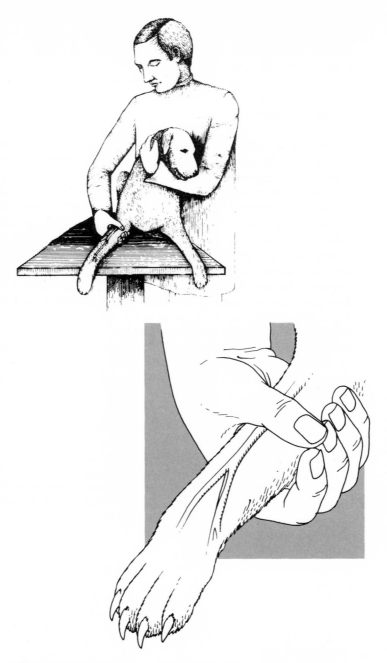

Fig. 21. Proper method of restraining the dog and raising the cephalic vein for venipuncture.

After preparing the syringe and wiping the injection site with alcohol, the anesthetist palpates the cephalic vein to check its position. If he has trouble finding it, gentle, rhythmic squeezing of the paw will further distend the vein.

The anesthetist's left hand is used to steady the limb at the injection site, and to pull the skin taut. The thumb can be placed beside the vein, in order to prevent its slipping away from the needle. Initial entry is made in the distal portion of the vein in order to allow sufficient room for threading the needle proximally into the vein or for further attempts at venipuncture if the initial attempt should fail.

Venipuncture consists of four movements which, in the hands of the skilled anesthetist, are so confluent that they appear as one: (1) with the bevel uppermost, the needle is pushed through the skin (Fig. 22A); (2) with the long axis of the needle nearly parallel to the long axis of the vein, the needle is depressed so that the point dimples the vein (Fig. 22B); (3) the needle is then advanced proximally into the vein (Fig. 22C); and (4) to ensure that the anesthetic agent will not enter any extravascular tissues, the needle is threaded along the vein for at least 1 cm (Fig. 22D). The syringe plunger is pulled back slightly, and if the needle has been correctly positioned blood should freely enter the syringe.

Fig. 22. Venipuncture.

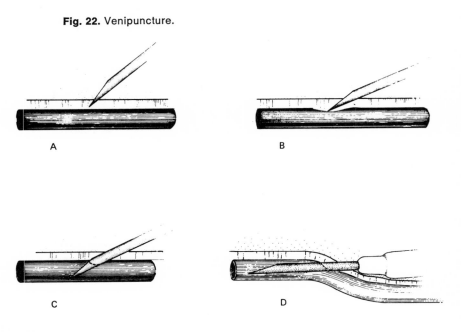

A

B

C

D

The needle hub and the syringe barrel are then secured to the limb with adhesive tape, applied in such a way that it does not obscure the syringe markings.

If barbiturate solutions are accidentally injected outside the blood vessels, the resulting vasospasm and the highly alkaline nature of the barbiturate may produce necrosis and subsequent sloughing of the skin. Infiltrating the area with a 2% solution of procaine in an amount approximately equal to the amount of barbiturate injected extravascularly will usually prevent this complication. If procaine is not readily available, sterile normal saline should be infiltrated into the area to dilute the anesthetic. Intra-arterial injections of barbiturates can cause spasm and endoarteritis, leading in some cases to loss of the limb.

B. Injection into other veins

Other injection sites that may be used for intravenous anesthesia are the saphenous, jugular, and sublingual veins.

For *saphenous venipuncture,* the patient should be restrained in the lateral recumbent position with all limbs extended. The vein is raised by pressure of the assistant's fingers circling the limb above the knee joint. The anesthetist grasps the tarsus and metatarsus in his left hand and immobilizes the vein by placing his thumb alongside it. The needle is inserted at the point where the vein crosses the tibia.

To make a *jugular venipuncture,* the assistant restrains the dog in an upright position at a height that is comfortable for the anesthetist. Then, by elevating the dog's chin, he stretches the neck and tenses the jugular vein. With the thumb or second finger of his left hand the anesthetist raises the vein by pressure on the neck at the level of the thoracic inlet; he then inserts the needle into the vein with the right hand.

Sublingual venipuncture is normally used in emergencies for the rapid administration of small quantities of drugs. The patient must be anesthetized or unconscious and lying in either the dorsal or the lateral recumbent position. The tongue is grasped with the left hand and pulled forward as far as it will come. Holding the tongue between the palm and the last three fingers, the anesthetist inserts his index finger under the tongue to raise the vein. He then immobilizes the vein between the thumb and the index finger while he makes the injection with a 25-gauge, $\frac{1}{2}$ inch needle. He inserts the needle to the hub, carefully guiding it into the vein. One should not attempt to aspirate blood, but should rely on vision and the sense of touch to determine when the vein has been entered. After withdrawing the needle, the thumb or a pledget of cotton should be held over the site of injection to minimize the formation of a hematoma.

C. Induction of anesthesia

Half of the calculated dose is injected rapidly, in order to take the dog through the excitement stage as quickly as possible. The anesthetist should then wait 2 to 3 minutes for blood–brain equilibrium to occur before he injects any more anesthetic. If the dog is in the excitement phase after this interval, half of the remaining anesthetic agent can be given. Thereafter, additional anesthetic is given in increments of 0.25 to 0.5 ml (allowing 2 or 3 minutes between each injection) until the stage of surgical anesthesia is reached. The syringe and needle should be left in position in case additional anesthesia is needed or in case it is necessary to give fluids or emergency drugs through the same needle.

III. Insertion of Endotracheal Tube

After the stage of surgical anesthesia is produced, an endotracheal tube should be inserted to prevent the aspiration of saliva and to permit positive-pressure ventilation in case artificial respiration becomes necessary. With the dog's neck extended, the tongue is pulled forward with a gauze sponge held in the fingers. Depressing the epiglottis with the larynogoscope blade pulls it forward, allowing visualization of the larynx and easy placement of the endotracheal tube. After the cuff of the endotracheal tube has been inflated with 5 ml of air, the chest should be compressed sharply but lightly. The resulting puff of air felt at the end of the tube indicates that it is in the correct position.

IV. Inhalation Anesthesia

Some highly volatile liquids, for example, ether, methoxyflurane, halothane, nitrous oxide, produce general anesthesia when sufficiently high concentrations of their vapors are inhaled. An inhalation anesthetic affects the nervous tissue by a reversible physical union with vital cellular substances. The central nervous system, because of its high vascularity and lipoidal content, is more susceptible than other systems of the body to the effects of an anesthetic.

When inhalation anesthesia is being administered it is important for the patient to receive a supply of oxygen. The exclusion of oxygen by strangulation by a deficiency in a closed-system anesthesia apparatus or by the inhalation of inert gases such as nitrogen or helium will cause asphyxia. This type of unconsciousness results in dangerous anoxemia, which is characterized clinically by a marked cyanosis. If the unconsciousness is produced by anesthesia, oxygen levels in the blood should be normal or above normal and cyanosis should be absent.

Oxygen should always be available for immediate administration in the event of asphyxiation or over dosage with inhalant or i.v. anesthetics. If adequate amounts of oxygen can be supplied to the brain, the animal can be kept alive while the tissues metabolize or eliminate the excess quantity of anesthetic.

A. Methods of administration

In general, inhalation anesthetics are administered by one of three basic methods: (1) open drop, (2) nonrebreathing, and (3) rebreathing.

In the *open-drop technique,* the anesthetic is dropped onto a gauze in a mask which is then placed over the dog's nose and mouth. As the patient breathes in, room air drawn through the gauze vaporizes the liquid. This method is simple and requires no specialized equipment, but it does not permit sensitive control over the depth of anesthesia.

In the *nonrebreathing (open) system* (Fig. 23A), the anesthesia is vaporized in a device which delivers the anesthetic to the patient. Normally, oxygen is flowed into the vaporizer and the resultant anesthetic–oxygen mixture is transported to the patient through rubber tubing. This can be attached to a face mask while anesthesia is being induced. After induction, an endotracheal tube is inserted and the rubber tubing is connected to it. The exhaled anesthetic mixture is released into the atmosphere.

The *rebreathing (closed) system* (Fig. 23B) employs a carbon-dioxide absorber as well as a vaporizer which may be in the rebreathing circuit or outside it. The exhaled anesthetic mixture flows through soda lime in the absorber which removes all of the carbon dioxide. This system is more efficient than the nonrebreathing system, because it uses less anesthetic and oxygen.

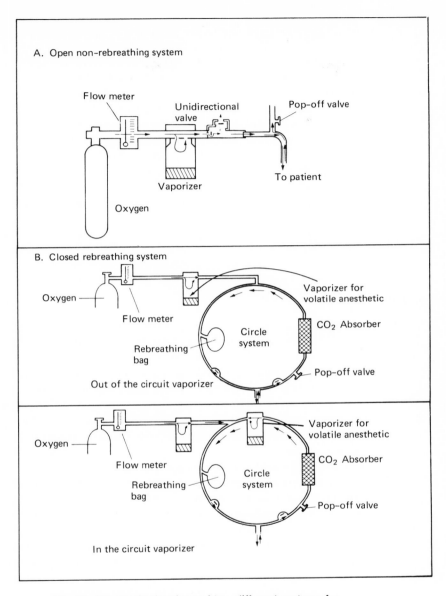

A. Open non-rebreathing system

Flow meter

Unidirectional valve

Pop-off valve

Vaporizer

To patient

Oxygen

B. Closed rebreathing system

Oxygen

Flow meter

Vaporizer for volatile anesthetic

CO_2 Absorber

Circle system

Rebreathing bag

Pop-off valve

Out of the circuit vaporizer

Oxygen

Flow meter

Vaporizer for volatile anesthetic

CO_2 Absorber

Circle system

Rebreathing bag

Pop-off valve

In the circuit vaporizer

Fig. 23. Schematic drawings of two different systems for administering volatile anesthetics. (A) Non-rebreathing (open) system. (B) Rebreathing (closed) systems. The upper picture shows a system with the vaporizer out of the circuit (VOC); the lower picture shows a VIC system, with the vaporizer in the circuit.

B. Volatile anesthetic agents

The inhalation anesthetics most commonly used for dogs are halothane and methoxyflurane. Both are potent, nonirritating, and nonexplosive.

Halothane, because of its high vaporization pressure, should never be used in an open system, but only in calibrated vaporizers. Halothane rapidly induces anesthesia when the inspired concentration reaches 3 to 5%. After the patient is anesthetized and intubated, anesthesia can be maintained with concentrations as low as 0.75 to 1.5%. Because of the rapid action of this gas, anesthetic levels can change very rapidly and lethal levels can be reached suddenly.

The cardiac and respiratory rates are good indicators of the depth of halothane anesthesia, and the anesthetist should observe them closely. Since the analgesic properties of halothane are weak, simultaneous administration of an analgesic may be necessary to eliminate the deep visceral reflexes.

Methoxyflurane has a very low vaporization pressure at room temperature (22°C), its maximum vaporization pressure being 3 to 3.5%. This agent is highly soluble in fat and other body tissues, which remove it from the blood and, thus, retard the build-up of anesthetic concentrations in the blood and brain. Because of the prolonged induction period with methoxyflurane, it is customary to induce anesthesia by the i.v. injection of an ultra-short-acting barbiturate and then maintain it with methoxyflurane. As a general rule, anesthetic concentrations should be maintained at approximately 3% for 15 to 20 minutes after intubation, to ensure that the depth of anesthesia is sufficient for surgery.

Methoxyflurane has very strong analgesic properties and often abolishes the palpebral, corneal, and pedal reflexes when the patient is still in the plane of light surgical anesthesia. It is difficult to build up lethal concentrations of methoxyflurane when the patient is breathing on his own. As anesthesia deepens, respiration usually slows down, thus, resulting in a decreased uptake of anesthetic. If respiratory arrest does occur, there is sufficient time to revive the patient by flushing the system with pure oxygen. If the patient is mechanically ventilated, however, lethal concentrations can be built up rapidly, making it imperative for the anesthetist constantly to monitor the animal's respiration and heart rate.

One drawback of methoxyflurane anesthesia is that it turns the blood cherry red, so that the relative stage of oxygenation cannot be gauged by the color of the blood.

V. Stages of Anesthesia

The neuromuscular reflexes are used as criteria for clinical classification of the depth of anesthesia. These reflexes can serve only as a guide, since they vary considerably in different animals and some of the signs may be absent with certain anesthetics. The central nervous system becomes depressed progressively through each of the clinical levels of anesthesia. During recovery from anesthesia, the dog passes through the same stages as during induction, but their order is reversed.

A. Stage I (stage of voluntary excitement)

Stages I and II are often referred to as the *period of induction.* In stage I there is analgesia without loss of consciousness, and the most characteristic features of this stage are excitement and struggling. The heart beats faster and stronger, and respirations are rapid and deep. The iris dilates as a result of the excitement, and urine and feces may be voided. Excessive salivation may be noted if the dog has not been given atropine. Regular administration of the anesthetic is difficult because of the dog's struggling.

B. Stage II (stage of involuntary excitement)

This stage begins when depression of the cortical centers leads to loss of consciousness and volitional control. The subconcious emotions (primarily the survival instinct) are the underlying cause of the dog's exaggerated reaction to external stimuli: reflex struggling, purposeless muscular movement, and sometimes whining or barking. Some dogs, however, show little reflex activity during this stage.

Respiration and pulse are influenced by the degree of excitement and exertion. As a rule, the pulse is rapid and strong. Commonly in the early part and sometimes throughout this stage, the respiration is uneven in depth and rate; breath holding may even occur. The eyelids are open wide and the irises are dilated because of sympathetic stimulation; they remain reactive to light, however. Reflex vomiting is common in this stage, unless food and water has been withheld for at least 6 hours or more before anesthesia.

Stage II may pass gradually into stage III or the dog may suddenly relax and appear to go into a deep sleep characterized by even, moderate breathing and a strong pulse. Stage II should be terminated as rapidly as possible, in order to reduce the hazard of injury to the anesthetist. If the anesthetic is administered too rapidly, however, there is danger of paralyzing the respiratory center by excessive concentrations of the agent.

C. Stage III (surgical anesthesia)

During this stage, the depressant action of the anesthesia is extended from the cortex and midbrain to the spinal cord. Consciousness, pain sensation, and spinal reflexes are abolished. Muscular relaxation occurs and coordinated movement disappears. Nearly all surgical procedures on dogs are done in this stage.

Surgical anesthesia is frequently divided into light and deep levels. In *light surgical anesthesia,* the eyelids remain open and random movement of the eyeball may occur, although the rate is slower than in stage II. Early in light surgical anesthesia, the iris constricts slightly so that it is only partially dilated; but with the approach of deep surgical anesthesia the iris dilates again.

The pedal (deep pain) reflex disappears almost at the onset of stage III. The corneal and palpebral reflexes are still present but are delayed. Muscle tone, which may be normal at the beginning of light surgical anesthesia, gradually decreases because of depression of the ordinary postural reflexes. Cutting of the skin or muscle does not cause reflex muscular contractions. The respiration becomes slow and regular and consists of both diaphragmatic and intercostal movements. Pulse and blood pressure are normal.

In deep surgical anesthesia, the lower reflexes (palpebral, corneal, and pedal) are completely abolished. Skeletal muscle tone rapidly disappears, leaving the dog flaccid. The irises are widely dilated. Feces may fall from the anus and some urine may escape from the urethra. The pulse is weak. Diaphragmatic respiration, although regular, gradually becomes more shallow. Intercostal respiration is depressed and begins to lag further and further behind the diaphragmatic respiration; when it disappears entirely, a dangerous depth of anesthetic depression has been reached. The failure of the *diaphragmatic* respiration indicates the beginning of stage IV.

Progressive paralysis of the hypothalamic centers during stage III inactivates the heat-regulating mechanism, so that loss of body heat fails to evoke such protective responses as shivering and vasoconstriction. Unless the patient is protected against heat loss, a marked fall in body temperature occurs.

D. Stage IV (medullary paralysis)

This stage is characterized by paralysis of the vital regulatory centers in the medulla. Respiratory arrest occurs and the blood pressure falls to the level of circulatory collapse. The heart usually beats weakly for a short time after respiration ceases. All reflexes are abolished, the irises are completely dilated, and the anal and urinary sphincters are completely relaxed. Unless artificial respiration is started immediately, death almost always results.

5

Water and Electrolyte Metabolism

WILLIAM J. WHITE AND C. MAX LANG

Certain diseases often lead to serious alterations in the water and electrolyte balance. It is easy to overlook the seriousness of these changes by failing to take into consideration the total amount of solute present. The concentration of solutes in body fluids is expressed as milligrams (or grams) per 100 ml, whereas the electrolyte concentration is expressed as milliequivalents per liter.

I. Evaluation of Disorders

A. Electrolyte imbalance

Even when the serum electrolytes are decreased, the electrolyte concentration is reduced only if the volume of extracellular fluid remains normal; if the total volume of fluid is reduced proportionately, this concentration can remain normal even with severe depletion of electrolytes. The reason is that the concentration is equal to the total amount of electrolyte present divided by the volume or weight of fluid in which it is dissolved.

As an example, let us suppose that a dog weighing 15 kg has a serum sodium concentration of 150 mEq/liter and an extracellular volume of 3.0 liters. Loss of sodium, with and without a simultaneous loss of extracellular water, would give the values shown in the following tabulation.

Unfortunately, it is not possible to measure accurately even the extracellular concentration of sodium and other electrolytes, far

	Plasma sodium (mEq/liter)	Extracellular water (liter)	Total extra-cellular sodium (mEq)
Initial values	150	3.0	450
Loss (10% Na, 0% water)	135	3.0	405
Loss (10% Na, 10% water)	150	2.7	405

less their intracellular concentration, which is the critical factor. It is within the cell that the metabolic processes of the body take place. Although direct measurement of electrolytes in the extracellular fluid is used as the basis for estimating the concentration of electrolytes in the intracellular fluid, there are often marked differences between intracellular and extracellular fluid composition.

Sodium is the principal cation and chloride is the principal anion of the extracellular fluids. All of the body chloride is essentially exchangeable, whereas a sizable quantity of sodium is exchanged slowly or not at all. This is the sodium of the bone, which constitutes about 40% of the total body sodium.

The principal cation of the intracellular fluids is potassium. Losses or gains of body potassium involve primarily the intracellular water. When a deficit in body potassium occurs for any reason, the potassium lost from the cells may be partially replaced by sodium, or there may be a compensatory loss of body cell mass, as in negative nitrogen balance. Conversely, a gain in body potassium can be associated with a loss of cellular sodium or an increase in body cell mass, as in positive nitrogen balance.

B. Acid–base imbalance

Another important consideration is the acid–base balance. The daily ingestion of acidic and basic salts leads to the production of large quantities of acid and some bases. To enable the body to maintain acid–base equilibrium, the newly produced acids are immediately buffered within the interstitial fluid, plasma, and red blood cells. The resultant quantities of acid are transferred to the lungs and kidneys for excretion.

The chemical buffers in the plasma and interstitial fluid include protein, bicarbonate, and inorganic phosphate. The cellular buffers include protein and organic phosphates. The buffering of blood is dependent upon a relatively rapid mechanism (involving the respiratory system and the red blood cells) and a relatively slow mechanism (involving the kidneys and tissue cells).

When the buffer systems of the body are not able to maintain a proper acid–base balance, the resultant change in the pH of the extracellular fluid causes further physiological disturbances. A blood pH above 7.45 indicates a state of alkalosis, and a pH below 7.35 indicates acidosis. (Alkalosis and acidosis are relative terms, since the body fluid seldom becomes truly acid.) The causes may be either metabolic (due to alterations in intake or to loss of bases or acids) or respiratory (caused by disturbances in the respiratory control of the carbon dioxide content of the blood).

Metabolic acidosis is a common disturbance of acid–base equilibrium. This condition occurs when there is an increase of acid or an excessive loss of base. The body tries to correct the resultant decrease in pH by stimulating pulmonary ventilation. As more carbon dioxide is eliminated, more is formed in the carbonic acid equilibrium by the combination of hydrogen and bicarbonate ions:

$$H^+ + HCO_3^- = H_2CO_3 = H_2O + CO_2$$

The result is a decrease in hydrogen ions and lowering of the P_{CO_2}. The decreased P_{CO_2}, however, eventually slows the rate of pulmonary ventilation and, in turn, the further correction of metabolic acidosis. Ultimate correction, therefore, depends upon increased excretion of acid by the kidney.

Metabolic alkalosis occurs less frequently than metabolic acidosis. It is usually associated with a loss of hydrogen ions, i.v. infusion of organic bases (for example, bicarbonate or citrate), or with a loss of chloride ions in excess of a corresponding loss of sodium ions. Any of these conditions results in an excess of basic anions which, in turn, increases the pH of the blood. The increased blood pH decreases pulmonary ventilation, causing the breathing to become shallow and slow, and the resultant retention of hydrogen ions causes the pH to return to normal. The decreased ventilation, however, also causes an increase in P_{CO_2}, which in turn stimulates the respiratory center. The final correction is dependent on the renal retention of hydrogen ions.

Respiratory acidosis results from increased carbon dioxide tension in the blood, which is due to interference with gaseous exchange, or hypoventilation. As the level of carbon dioxide increases in the blood, it causes a shift in the carbonic acid equilibrium, with a resultant increase in hydrogen ions. The body compensates by renal excretion of hydrogen ions and nonbicarbonate anions to produce a more acid urine. Also, it conserves bicarbonate ions by excreting chloride ions. Respiratory alkalosis is induced by prolonged hyperventilation, which results in a plasma carbonic-acid deficit. Hyperventilation can be caused by anxiety, fever, anoxia, or stimulation of the respiratory center by drugs or disease. As a result of hyperventilation, the carbonic acid equilibrium shifts to an increased production of carbon dioxide. In order to conserve hydrogen ions that are being used as a result of this shift, renal excretion of bicarbonate ions is increased. There is also a concomitant increase in the retention of hydrogen ions and nonbicarbonate anions by the renal tubules.

C. Dehydration

Water plays an essential role in electrolyte metabolism and acid–base balance. Too much or too little water in the body cells may lead to cellular dysfunction and even to death. The major causes of fluid depletion are diarrhea, vomiting, hemorrhage, gross tissue damage, and starvation. Warm-blooded animals constantly eliminate water from the body—both through the respiratory tract and skin (in the dissipation of body heat) and from the urinary tract (in the elimination of urea salts and other end products of metabolism). Since this elimination of water continues regardless of the water intake, the animal whose fluid intake is inadequate becomes progressively dehydrated. Dehydration is hastened by fever, sweating, or diuresis, as well as by vomiting or diarrhea.

Clinically, dehydration may be assessed by a variety of signs (Table I). With severe dehydration, skin turgor and ocular tension are greatly reduced, the buccal mucosa is dry and wrinkled, capillary-filling time is prolonged, the pulse is sluggish, and the extremities are cold. Skin turgor is probably the most commonly used sign, since the skin and muscle are the principal body depots of reserve water. Under conditions of dehydration, the skin gives up a greater portion of its water than any other tissue.

Among the laboratory tests to assessing the severity of dehydration (Table I), the hematocrit and hemoglobin are the ones most commonly used because of the ease in making these determinations. An increase of 25% in the hematocrit is usually attended by grave signs and clinical manifestations of a very severe dehydration. When the hematocrit increases to 40% or more above normal, death usually follows.

Table I Signs of dehydration

	Mild (4%[1])	Moderate (6%[1])	Severe (8% or more[1])
Elasticity of skin	Normal to slightly reduced	Markedly reduced	Absent or very severely reduced
Mucous membranes	Little perceptible change	Dryness of surface with noticeable decrease	Extensive dryness and congestion; lack of normal secretions
Appearance of eyes	Normal	Sunken	Very sunken; intraocular pressure decreased
Thirst	Present	More severe	Severe, but patient may have difficulty drinking
Haircoat	Dry and disheveled	Dry and disheveled	Dry and disheveled
Urine			
Volume	Slight decrease[2]	Absent or decrease[3]	Severe oliguria[4] or anuria
Electrolytes and protein concentration	Slight increase[2]	Moderate increase[3]	Marked increase[4]
Specific gravity	Slight increase[2]	Moderate increase[3]	Very severe increase (>1.030)
Hematocrit and hemoglobin			
Concentration	Slight increase[2]	Moderate increase[3]	Marked increase[4]
Serum electrolytes and other chemical constituents	Slight increase[2]	Moderate increase[3]	Marked increase[4]

[1] Water loss expressed as a percentage of body weight.

[2] Ten to 20% above or below normal values.

[3] Twenty to 40% above or below normal values.

[4] More than 40% above or below normal values.

II. Replacement Therapy

The goal of fluid therapy is to correct deficits and imbalances of fluids and electrolytes, and to prevent further depletions without creating new imbalances. In order to determine whether fluid therapy is needed and what type to use, the patient's condition must be accurately assessed on the basis of a thorough physical examination and appropriate clinical laboratory data. The importance of the physical examination cannot be overemphasized. Although laboratory analyses are necessary to assess the type of imbalance present and the success of therapy, their immediate value is limited because they relate to the state of the patient in the past.

A. Routes of administration

Fluids and electrolytes for replacement therapy may be administered by mouth (per os), by rectum, or parenterally (intravenously, subcutaneously, or intraperitoneally).

Each route has its own advantages and limitations. The route of choice is the one whose advantages match the requirement for treatment and the characteristics of the fluid to be administered.

1. *Oral*

The gastrointestinal tract is the most physiological route for the administration of water, electrolytes, and nutritional substances. In health, it functions well without regard for the pH, composition, toxicity, or volume of the solution. The oral route is preferred over all others, except when it is ruled out by disease of the gastrointestinal tract or when the condition demands a more rapid rate of administration. After acute defects have been corrected by parenteral therapy, it is often possible to complete the replenishment of water, electrolytes, and nutrients by normally administered fluids.

2. *Intravenous*

Of all the routes mentioned, the vein is probably the most versatile and the most dangerous. Because the solutions are placed directly into the circulation, continual clinical evaluation of the patient is necessary. When administration is prolonged, or hypertonic solutions are used, the concentration of electrolytes in the blood must be monitored frequently.

The rate of i.v. administration is also an important factor. Isotonic solutions of electrolytes or mixtures of isotonic electrolyte solutions with 5% dextrose should be given at the rate of 3 to 6 ml pound/hour. More rapid administration can result in pulmonary edema by increasing the pressure in the systemic veins, chambers of the heart, and pulmonary vessels, thus, overdistending them and reducing the effect of osmotic pressure of the plasma. For this reason, frequent auscultation of the chest is important when fluids are being administered i.v.

3. *Subcutaneous*

Fluids can be administered subcutaneously by injecting them into the loose connective tissue which attaches the dermis to the underlying organs. The skin of many animals—the dog, for example—is rather loosely attached, thus, allowing for free skin movement and increasing the capacity of the subcutaneous tissues to accept a large volume of extracellular fluid with little rise in tissue pressure.

The rate at which subcutaneously administered fluid is absorbed depends upon the size of the absorbing surface (capillary wall) exposed to the fluid. Any factor which reduces the surface or the blood flow through the capillary decreases the rate of absorption. The rate of absorption can be increased by the use of multiple injection sites, and the exclusion of vasoconstricting drugs.

Because the rate of absorption of subcutaneously administered fluids depends on tissue perfusion and the osmotic pressure of the blood, there is no danger that rapid expansion of the blood volume will lead to pulmonary edema. This route of administration is therefore much safer than the i.v. route. Subcutaneous fluid therapy, however, does have some very definite limitations:

a. The solution should be isotonic and balanced with respect to major plasma ionic constituents, e.g., sodium and chloride. Under no circumstances should the solution be sodium-free. Such unbalanced solutions may increase the existing sodium depletion by causing a migration of sodium into the subcutaneous fluids.

b. The solution should not be hypertonic (for example, 50% dextrose), nor should it contain molecules with a high molecular weight (for example, dextran, albumin, or plasma protein). Such solutions tend to absorb water from the surrounding tissues and the plasma until they have become isotonic with plasma; only then are they slowly absorbed into the bloodstream.

c. The solution should be free of highly irritating chemicals such as ammonium chloride, calcium chloride, or concentrated solutions of amino acids.

4. *Intraperitoneal*

Intraperitoneal administration of fluid leads to more rapid absorption than the subcutaneous route, but otherwise has the same limiting factors. In addition, it is not so easy to monitor the fate of the fluid given intraperitoneally. The possibility of peritonitis always exists, and puncture of visceral organs is not uncommon.

B. Types and amounts of fluids

1. *For electrolyte and fluid imbalance*

Discussions of the types and amounts of fluids that should be administered in various clinical situations are available in a number of texts. As a general rule, one should attempt to calculate the amounts of electrolytes and fluids the animal has lost and then select the replacement fluid and the route of administration best suited to correct the deficit. The amount needed may be determined by the following calculations:

1. Electrolyte deficit (mEq/liter) = normal serum concentration (mEq/liter) — patient's serum concentration (mEq/liter).
2. Extracellular fluid volume (liters) = body weight (kilograms) $\times$ 0.20
3. Total deficit (mEq) = deficit per liter $\times$ extracellular fluid volume (liters)
4. Volume of solution required (ml) =
$$\frac{\text{total deficit (mEq)}}{\text{electrolyte solution (mEq/liter)}} \times 100 \text{ ml/liter}$$

2. *For nutrition*

In many cases, parenteral fluid therapy is used not only to correct fluid and electrolyte imbalance but also to provide parenteral nutrition. It should be remembered, however, that a few hundred milliliters of commercially prepared carbohydrate, or protein solution do not come close to fulfilling an animal's nutritional requirements. Such solutions should be used only to support the animal for a short time, until other forms of nutrition can be administered by stomach tube or until the animal starts eating.

The carbohydrate most commonly used for parenteral feeding is glucose. Glucose provides approximately 4 Cal per gram. When given i.v., glucose is oxidized by the body to yield energy, converted to glycogen for later use, or converted to body fat. The maximum rate of i.v. administration that can be tolerated by most species is 0.5 to 0.9 gm/kg of body weight per hour.

Protein can be provided as protein hydrolysate, which is prepared from casein by the hydrolytic action of hydrochloric acid. It is usually combined with dextrose to ensure that the amino acids will not be diverted to the energy pool by deamination. In most commercial solutions the concentration of protein hydrolysate is only 5%, although solutions containing as much as 38 gm/1000 ml are available. Protein hydrolysate solutions may be given orally or intravenously, but their utilization is better if they are given by the oral route. If protein hydrolysate is given too rapidly by vein, it will cause chills, fever, nausea and vomiting—probably because of the glutamic acid contained in the hydrolysate. The optimum rate of i.v. injection is less than 12 ml/minute.

The normal protein requirement of most animals is assumed to be 1 gm/kilogram of body weight/day. If the animal is in a negative nitrogen balance, 2 gm/kg should be given daily until a positive nitrogen balance is established. Approximately twice this amount of glucose should be given simultaneously to avoid deamination.

In summary, fluid therapy should not be attempted until the animal's electrolytes, pH, and energy requirements have been thoroughly evaluated. Because our knowledge is still inadequate to permit absolute precision in prescribing fluids and electrolytes, we have to rely on the body to compensate for minor therapeutic errors or deficiencies. If renal function is adequate and if all necessary electrolytes are supplied in approximately the required amounts, the body itself will, in most cases, make the final adjustment.

Surgical Procedures

The surgical procedures discussed in this section are selected to demonstrate basic principles of physiology and to correlate with the other basic-science courses in the first-year medical curriculum. This correlation will depend largely, of course, on the clinical chemistry tests that are carried out during the postoperative period. These are discussed in Part III.

6

Laparotomy

C. MAX LANG

Laparotomy (Gk. *lapara,* flank and Gk. *tomē,* a cutting) is defined by Dorland[1] as a "surgical incision through the flank: less correctly, but more generally, abdominal section at any point." This operation is fundamental to all abdominal surgery.

I. Anatomic Descriptions

Topographic anatomical terms are used to indicate precisely the position and direction of parts of the body. The surgeon must have a thorough understanding of these terms in order to follow the procedure and to communicate with his team members. In this procedure, and the others in this text, the terms are used as if the dog were in a normal standing position.

The **ventral** surface is that directed toward the plane of support and the opposite surface is **dorsal.** The head end of the animal is called **cranial** (anterior), and the tail end **caudal** (posterior). If the body is divided into equal halves by a longitudinal plane, a structure or object that is nearer to it than another is called **medial.** Likewise, a structure or object which is further than another from the median plane is **lateral** to it. These terms are similar in use to proximal and distal. However, these latter terms

[1] Dorland's *Illustrated Medical Dictionary.* (1974). 25th ed. Philadelphia: W. B. Saunders Company.

are used in reference to a particular structure or other point of reference rather than of the median plane. **Proximal** is closer to that point of reference and **distal** is further away.

Positioning of the animal on the operating table is usually described with a topographic anatomical term followed by the word **recumbency.** The anatomical term is the surface of the animal that is placed against the operating table. For example, if a dog is placed on its back, it is referred to as dorsal recumbency.

II. Surgical Procedure

The anesthetized, prepared animal is placed on the operating table in the dorsal recumbent position, and the legs are tied. Antiseptic solution is applied first to the proposed incision line, and then alternately working outward on each side of this line until the entire shaved area has been swabbed. The swab is then discarded into the kick bucket. This procedure should be repeated three more times, each time with a clean swab saturated with antiseptic solution.

The patient is draped so that the incision site is left undraped in the center of the field (Fig. 24). If the drape does not have a precut hole in its center, this must be done after the drape is in place. The surgeon establishes the correct plane for the incision site by palpating, through the drape sheet, the xiphoid process and the symphysis pubis. He then tents the drape sheet over the proposed incision site and cuts a hole with a pair of Mayo scissors. The sterile drape is secured to the skin with four Backhaus towel clamps placed in such a manner as to avoid bunching.

A. Making the incision

In dogs, the best site for an abdominal incision is the midline. In human patients, on the other hand, the midline incision is confined almost entirely to gynecologic surgery, where the incision is below the umbilicus. Because the aponeurosis above the umbilicus is so thin and friable in human beings, the linea alba is avoided whenever possible.

If the abdominal incision is made exactly on the midline, it will transect the ventral abdominal fascia along the linea alba. The linea alba is a junction of the fascial sheaths of the abdominal musculature. Therefore, the only tissue layer directly beneath the linea alba is the peritoneum. Because the linea alba is often difficult to locate, most midline incisions are slightly lateral to it. These

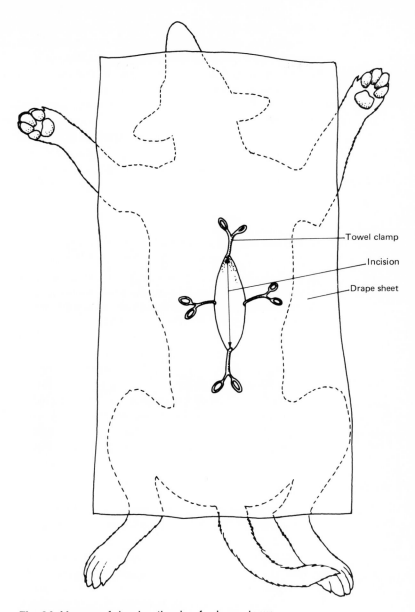

Towel clamp

Incision

Drape sheet

Fig. 24. Manner of draping the dog for laparotomy.

are called *paramedian* incisions. It differs from a true midline incision in that the rectus abdominis muscle will be between the ventral abdominal fascia and the peritoneum.

The skin incision should be made with one stroke of a #10 blade inserted in a #4 handle. This incision should be with the curved edge and not the tip of the blade. The only tissues cut should be the skin and the superficial subcutaneous tissue (Fig. 25A). Because of the possibility of contamination, the scalpel and blade used for the skin incision should not be used again during the procedure.

The incision should begin approximately 3 cm below the xiphoid and extend caudally for 10 to 15 cm depending on the length of the dog. The longer the incision, the greater force will be required to appose the edges. If the incision is too short, how-

Fig. 25. The laparotomy incision. (A) Incision of the skin and subcutaneous tissue reveals the ventral abdominal fascia. (B) After the ventral abdominal fascia has been incised, the rectus abdominis muscle can be seen. (C) The rectus abdominis muscle fibers are separated by blunt dissection to reveal the peritoneum. (D) The peritoneum is raised with forceps before being nicked with a scalpel. (E) The relationship of structures in the midline incision site.

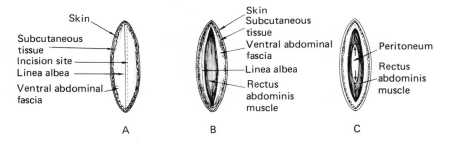

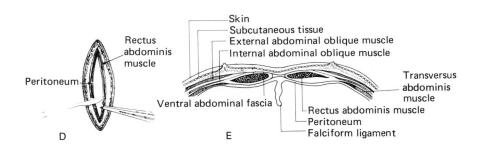

ever, rough handling of the tissues will be required. A long incision will heal as quickly as a short one, since healing occurs from side to side rather than from end to end.

Macroscopic arteries and veins severed in making the incision are tied with 000 surgical gut. A small amount of blood from microscopic vessels is normal. If excessive, this bleeding can be controlled by applying firm pressure on the area with a dry sponge. Tissue surrounding the smaller bleeders may be clamped with hemostats until bleeding has stopped. However, to minimize trauma, the surgeon should try to clamp as little of the surrounding tissue as possible.

The exposed subcutaneous tissue should then be bluntly dissected with Metzenbaum dissection scissors to expose the ventral abdominal fascia. A sterile scalpel (#3 handle, #10 blade) is used to make a small paramedian incision in the fascia, approximately at the center of the proposed opening (Fig. 25B). Care should be taken to avoid cutting the rectus abdominis muscle. A grooved director is then inserted into this opening, and the scalpel is used to complete the incision longitudinally in both directions, thus, exposing the rectus abdominis muscle. Allis tissue forceps are placed on the incised edge of the ventral abdominal fascia to hold the incision open.

Dissection through the rectus abdominis muscle is achieved by inserting a closed hemostat into the muscle tissue and opening it along the line of the muscle fibers (Fig. 25C). The incision is extended by using two closed hemostats pulled in opposite directions in the line of the muscle fibers. When the opening is large enough, the hemostats are replaced by fingers and the incision is completed by pulling the muscle apart, in the line of its fibers, to the length of the incision in the abdominal ventral fascia.

Any incision can develop *dead space* if there is any significant amount of tissue separation adjacent to the incision. If these spaces are not reunited with sutures (00 chromic surgical gut) they will fill with tissue fluids. This puts additional pressure on the healing incision and may serve as a growth medium for bacteria.

To ensure that no viscera are cut when the peritoneum is incised, forceps are used to lift the peritoneum before nicking it with the scalpel (Fig. 25D). The incision is extended by placing a grooved director under the fascia and pushing with Metzenbaum dissection scissors.

The incision in the peritoneum should be made lateral to the linea alba and should be closed separately to provide extra strength and to reduce the possibility of adhesions.

B. Exploring the abdominal cavity

After the skin edges are covered with moist sterile sponges, a Balfour retaining retractor is inserted into the opening to provide adequate exposure during exploration of the abdominal cavity.

After the abdominal cavity is opened, a lacy appearing structure, called the greater omentum, is seen. The greater omentum is an empty, double-walled sac of connective tissue, extending from the greater curvature of the stomach to the urinary bladder. To reach the underlying structures, the surgeon simply grasps it with his fingers and pulls it cranially until its caudal and lateral margins are free from the intestines. No attempt should be made to reposition the greater omentum after the procedure is completed.

The falciform ligament (Fig. 25E), located immediately to the side of the incision or within the incision itself, extends from the umbilicus to the liver, and the spleen is lateral and adjacent to the greater curvature of the stomach (Fig. 26). By following the curvature of the stomach in a caudal direction, the duodenum and pancreas can be identified, along with the jejunum and ileum. The mesentery and the mesenteric lymph nodes can be seen by gently picking up the small intestines.

The common bile duct lies to the right of the hepatic artery and inferior to the portal vein; it opens into the duodenum about 2.5 to 5 cm from the pylorus. If it is not readily visible, it may be necessary to feel for the firm, tubelike structure of the bile duct in the mesenteric tissues adjacent to the duodenum and follow it in a retrograde direction.

The urinary bladder is located in the most caudal aspect of the abdominal cavity. Just dorsal to the urinary bladder is the descending loop of the colon. The transverse and ascending colon, as well as the ileum and cecum, are easily recognized. The ileocecal valve can be palpated near the junction of the ileum and the colon.

A laparotomy sponge moistened with warm normal saline is used to push the intestines to the right side of the abdominal cavity so that kidney, ureter, and renal blood vessels on the left side can be identified. The adrenal gland and its blood vessels are located medial to the anterior pole of the kidney. Medial to the adrenals are the inferior vena cava and the abdominal aorta. The pulse in this vessel should be checked and recorded.

The saline sponge is then removed and used to pack the intestines on the left side, so that the kidneys, adrenals, and blood vessels on the right side can be located. The right adrenal gland may be under the vena cava and its location identified by gentle

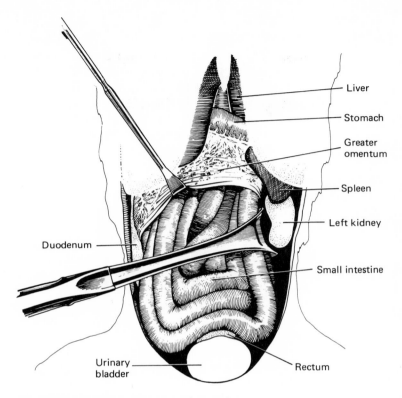

Fig. 26. Abdominal viscera, ventral aspect.

palpation. When all of the abdominal organs have been identified, the surgeon removes the sponges and checks the abdominal cavity for any sponges or instruments that may have been left in the area.

C. Closing the incision

After gently adjusting the organs to their normal positions, the surgeon grasps each cut edge of the peritoneum with Allis tissue forceps placed opposite each other. Bringing the peritoneum slightly out of the incision by gentle traction, he closes it with a simple continuous suture pattern using a tapered (or atraumatic) curved needle threaded with 00 chromic surgical gut (Fig. 27A). If the falciform ligament was in the incision site, it must be removed before closing the peritoneum by cutting it free.

The same needle and the same type of surgical gut are used to close the ventral abdominal fascia with simple interrupted sutures

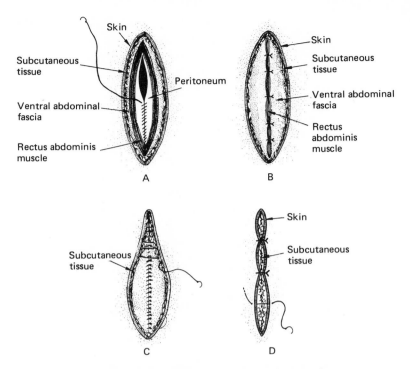

Fig. 27. Closure of the abdominal incision. The peritoneum is closed with a simple continuous suture (A); the ventral abdominal fascia, with simple interrupted sutures (B); the subcutaneous tissue, with a simple continuous suture (C); and the skin with simple interrupted sutures (D).

(Fig. 27B) placed so that there is no sagging of the wound edges. This objective is best accomplished by placing the first suture in the center of the incision, and subsequent sutures in the center of each remaining space until the incision is closed. Sutures should be approximately 0.5 cm apart. Knots should be tied so that there is minimum tension and maximum apposition (without bunching) of the wound edges. The ventral abdominal fascia, being the strongest of these soft tissues, is relied upon to prevent wound dehiscence.

Subcutaneous sutures (Fig. 27C) make final closure easier and enhance the strength and neatness of the resulting scar. Simple interrupted or continuous sutures of 0 or 00 plain gut placed in the subcutaneous tissues help to appose the skin edges, obliterate dead space, and minimize wound gapping.

The skin is closed with simple interrupted sutures of nonabsorbable suture material threaded on a straight or curved needle (Fig. 27D). When the last suture is placed the apposing edges should be gently pressed together wth a sterile sponge. The drapes are then removed and the incision may be covered with a sterile spray bandage.

III. Postsurgical Care

The student team is responsible for the patient until the sutures have been removed (7 to 10 days after surgery) and all laboratory procedures are completed. During this period of time the following observations should be made and recorded legibly on the patient's record B.I.D. (*bis in die*—twice a day):

1. Rectal temperature
2. Respiratory rate
3. Approximate food and water intake
4. Approximate amount of urine and feces
5. Behavior and general condition
6. Description of wound

The recorded data should be initialed by the team member making the observations. Responsibility for his patients will become a way of life to the medical student and should take precedence over all other activities.

IV. Laboratory Procedures

On the second postoperative day a blood sample is collected and submitted to the laboratory. This sample should be accompanied by the appropriate form requesting (1) a white blood cell count, (2) a differential count, (3) the hemoglobin, and (4) the hematocrit. It will be the student's responsibility to make a preliminary analysis of these data.

7

Splenectomy

C. MAX LANG

Splenectomy (Gk. *splēn,* spleen and Gk. *ektomē,* excision) is defined by Dorland[1] as "excision or extirpation of the spleen." Experimental removal of the spleen affords the student surgeon experience in vascular ligation and demonstrates the vasoconstrictive action of a sympathomimetic drug (epinephrine) on the spleen.

I. Spleen

A. Anatomy

In the dog, the spleen lies along the greater curvature of the stomach in the left hypogastric region. The location is dependent on the size and position of the other abdominal organs—particularly the stomach, to which it is loosely attached. The spleen has a thick trabecular framework and is firm in consistency, especially when contracted. When relaxed, it is sigmoid in shape and the ventral end, or free extremity, lies on the floor of the abdominal cavity, sometimes extending across the ventral midline to the right side.

The main blood supply to the spleen (Fig. 28) is furnished by the splenic artery, which is a branch of the celiac artery. In the dog, the splenic artery divides into approximately 25 branches, all

[1] Dorland's *Illustrated Medical Dictionary.* (1974). 25th ed. Philadelphia: W. B. Saunders Company.

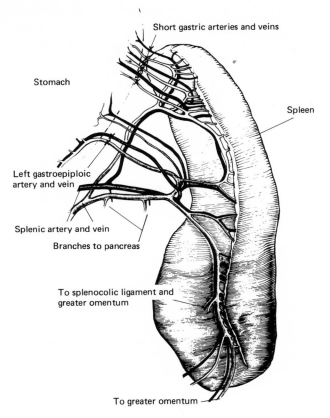

Short gastric arteries and veins

Stomach

Spleen

Left gastroepiploic
artery and vein

Splenic artery and vein

Branches to pancreas

To splenocolic ligament and
greater omentum

To greater omentum

Fig. 28. The canine spleen and its blood supply. The arteries
are shown in black, the veins in white.

of which pass through the long hilus. Blood from the spleen
drains into the splenic vein and thence into the gastrosplenic vein.

True accessory spleens are uncommon in the dog. When present,
they are usually the result of postnatal trauma.

The capsule of the spleen in the dog, and in many other lower
animals, is a smooth muscle sac of great strength. In these animals,
sympathetic stimulation results in intense contraction of the splenic
capsule, whereas sympathetic inhibition results in considerable
splenic relaxation, thus, providing for storage of blood. Although
the splenic capsule in man is nonmuscular, dilatation of the vessels
within the spleen allows the storage of several hundred milliliters
of blood, most of which is released when the vessels constrict under
the influence of sympathetic stimulation.

B. Physiology

The spleen filters the blood and removes the wornout erythrocytes from the circulation. From these cells it produces bilirubin, which is subsequently collected by the liver. The reticuloendothelial cells of the spleen ingest the released hemoglobin and the cell stroma, extract the iron from the ingested hemoglobin, and release it into the blood, to be used again by the bone marrow in the production of new erythrocytes.

The reticuloendothelial cells of the spleen also remove debris, bacteria, and parasites from the blood. In many infectious diseases, the spleen enlarges in order to accomplish this cleansing function more adequately. The white pulp that fills much of the spleen is actually a large accumulation of lymphocytes. In addition to producing many of the body's lymphocytes, the spleen also produces most of the monocytes in the circulation and plays an important role in the production of antibodies.

II. Surgical Procedure

The incision for this procedure is the same as that described for the laparotomy (Chapter 6). The incision should be long enough to allow the spleen to be withdrawn from the abdominal cavity but it need not extend caudal to the umbilicus. After lifting the spleen out of the abdomen with moistened sponges, identify the splenic vessels in the gastrosplenic ligament (splenic portion of the greater omentum). These vessels will be more visible in the side containing less fat. After identifying the splenic artery by its pulsation, dissect the portion to be injected and ligate from its surrounding tissue. This gentle blunt dissection should be parallel to the direction of the splenic artery to avoid accidental tearing. Ligatures of 00 silk should then be preplaced approximately 1 cm above and below the anticipated injection site. The surgeon then slowly injects 2 ml of a 1:1000 solution of epinephrine into the splenic artery. If the epinephrine is injected too rapidly, violent contraction of the spleen will result.

The splenic artery is then double-ligated with the preplaced sutures and severed between the two distal ligatures. Any aberrant arteries are similarly ligated. Thus deprived of its blood supply, the spleen maintains the contraction produced by the epinephrine. The veins are then double-ligated with 00 silk and severed between the ligatures. All vessels should be ligated as close to the spleen as possible, in order to preserve the gastrosplenic omentum. Ligatures on the splenic side can be cut short; those on the stomach side are left long.

After all the vessels have been ligated, the spleen is removed and the long ends of the ligatures are tied together (Fig. 29A) in groups of 2 to 4 vessels. A few inverting sutures placed in the

Fig. 29. Completion of splenectomy. (A) The vessels on the stomach side are ligated with long sutures, which are tied together after the spleen has been removed. (B) The omental stump is then inverted and sutured to prevent adhesions.

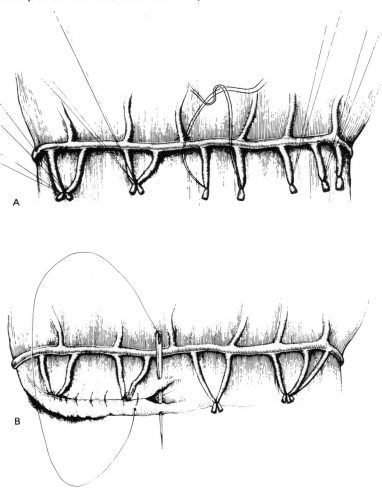

stump of omentum (Fig. 29B) will create a smooth surface and thereby reduce the size and number of adhesions.

After inspecting the abdominal cavity for any abnormalities or signs of bleeding, the surgeon closes the incision in the manner previously described (Chapter 6).

III. Postsurgical Care

Basic postoperative care is the same as that described in the preceding chapter. If healing occurs normally, the skin sutures can be removed in seven to ten days.

IV. Clinical Considerations

The most common indication for removal of the spleen is the presence of a tumor. Traumatic rupture of the spleen is another frequent indication for splenectomy.

In spite of its seemingly important role, the spleen does not appear to be essential to life, or even to health. In its absence, most of its normal functions are taken over by other tissues.

After splenectomy, a mild leukocytosis and thrombocytosis may persist for months, and nucleated erythrocytes and red corpuscles containing Howell–Jolly bodies may be present in the blood for years. Although these findings are of interest, people without their spleens can live a normal life span with no apparent impairment of their health.

8

Lobectomy

WILLIAM J. WHITE AND C. MAX LANG

Thoracotomy (Gk *thōrax*, breastplate and Gk. *tomē*, a cutting) refers to the process of surgically incising the chest, and pneumonectomy (Gk. *pneumōn*, lung and Gk. *ektomē*, excision) to the process of removing a lung. In clinical practice, however, pneumonectomy is rare.[1] The lung operation performed most commonly is a lobectomy (Gk. *lobos*, lobe and Gk. *ektomē*, excision) or the removal of a single lobe of the lung.[1] In occasional cases, small segments of a lobe are excised for therapeutic or diagnostic purposes.

The experimental removal of the left diaphragmatic lobe of the lung affords the student surgeon experience in working with thoracic viscera and helps to give him an appreciation of the respiratory mechanisms which operate to maintain normal gas concentrations and a normal pH in the blood.

I. Lungs

A. Anatomy

The lungs are distinctly lobed structures. Each lung is divided into apical, cardiac, and diaphragmatic lobes, and the right lung has a fourth lobe—the intermediate—which lies dorsocaudal to the

---

[1] Dorland's *Illustrated Medical Dictionary.* (1974). 25th ed. Philadelphia: W. B. Saunders Co.

heart. The lobes are separated by deep fissures which completely divide the parenchyma of the lungs. In the dog the only exception is the fissure between the left apical and the left cardiac lobe, which only partially separates the two.

The bronchial tree begins at the bifurcation of the trachea, which forms the right and left pulmonary bronchi. At the hilus of the lung each pulmonary bronchus divides into lobar bronchi, each of which supplies a different lobe. Within each lobe, the lobar bronchus divides into several segmental or tertiary bronchi. These segmental bronchi then divide dichotomously into several orders of bronchioles, which eventually divide into respiratory bronchioles and finally into pulmonary alveoli.

The pulmonary arteries carry nonaerated blood from the right ventricle of the heart to the lungs for gaseous exchange. About 4 cm from its origin in the conus arteriosus of the right ventricle, the pulmonary trunk bifurcates to form the right and left pulmonary arteries.

The right pulmonary artery leaves the pulmonary trunk and courses to the right for about 2 cm before giving off a branch to the right apical lobe. About 1 cm beyond this branch, the artery divides into several vessels supplying the cardiac, diaphragmatic, and intermediate lobes on the right side. The left pulmonary artery is shorter and smaller in diameter than the right. It divides into two or more branches, one of which enters the left apical lobe, the other(s) enter the bulk of the lung before subdividing to supply the cardiac and diaphragmatic lobes.

Ordinarily, each lobe is drained by one pulmonary vein. These veins usually enter individually into the dorsum of the left atrium, but it is not uncommon for the veins from the diaphragmatic lobes to fuse with veins draining other lobes.

B. Physiology

In vertebrates, such as the dog, the respiratory and cardiovascular (circulatory) systems together provide a mechanism for the exchange and transport of oxygen and carbon dioxide between the cells of the body and the external environment. Muscular contraction of the thorax mechanically pumps air in and out of the lungs. Blood containing gases from cellular respiration is transported to and from the lungs by the circulatory system. In the lungs, the blood gases and atmospheric gases are exchanged across the semipermeable membrane of the alveolar capillary.

The function of both the respiratory and the circulatory system is controlled by the respiratory center located in the medulla. An elaborate chemoreceptor mechanism monitors the gaseous makeup of the blood and relays this information to the respiratory center.

Venous blood, having an oxygen tension (p_{O_2}) of 35 to 45 Torr and a carbon dioxide (p_{CO_2}) tension of 44 to 48 Torr, is equilibrated in the lungs with humidified inspired air, which has a p_{O_2} of 160 Torr and a p_{CO_2} of less than 1 Torr. Following exchange, the blood leaving the lungs has a p_{O_2} of 90 to 100 Torr and a p_{CO_2} of 35 to 40 Torr; the exhaled gas has a p_{O_2} of 120 Torr and a p_{CO_2} of 30 Torr.

It is not simply the amount of air entering the lungs (ventilation) that determines the partial pressures (tensions) of oxygen and carbon dioxide in the blood, but rather the combined effects of ventilation and perfusion. Not all areas of the lung are ventilated or perfused to the same degree; thus, blood entering the left ventricle from one area of the lungs may have a higher p_{O_2} and a lower p_{CO_2} than blood from another area. As blood from all areas of the lung is admixed in the left atrium, the final p_{O_2} and p_{CO_2} of the arterial blood is produced.

During normal activity, as little as 50% of the total pulmonary capacity may be needed to maintain a normal arterial p_{O_2} and p_{CO_2}. The remaining 50% of the lung serves as a reserve for use during periods of increased activity. In order to prevent atelectasis and to maintain the viability of the tissue, vascular and gaseous shunting mechanisms route blood and inspired gas to these reserve areas during periods of inactivity as well as during strenuous exercise.

Many factors (ambient temperature, neurogenic stimuli, anesthesia, exercise, disease, etc.) may alter the ratio of ventilation to perfusion for varying periods of time. Under such conditions, the p_{O_2} and p_{CO_2} (and hence the pH) of the blood may be significantly altered. Sometimes the shunting mechanisms alone are not enough to restore the normal gas composition of the blood, and pharmacological or surgical intervention becomes necessary. In many cases the blood buffers and renal excretion of fixed acid or base can cope with these blood–gas imbalances except during periods of increased activity. In such cases these deficiencies show up clinically as exercise intolerance.

II. Surgical Procedure

To remove the left diaphragmatic lobe of the lung, the dog is placed in the right lateral recumbent position, with the left foreleg in full extension (Fig. 30). Depending on the conformation of the

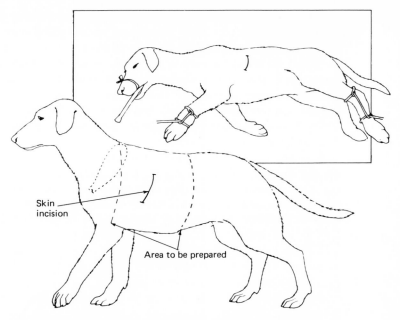

Fig. 30. Diagram of the dog showing the incision site and the area to be prepared for a left thoracotomy. The insert shows a dog in the right lateral recumbent position.

dog, it may be necessary to place a pad between the thorax and the operating table in order to elevate and tense the thorax. The dog should be clipped from the cranial thorax to the last rib and from the dorsal to the ventral midline.

A. Opening the chest

After the area has been scrubbed, disinfected, and draped, a curved incision at least 12 cm in length should be made in the fifth intercostal space with a #20 blade attached to a #4 handle. The skin incision (Fig. 30) should be made 3 to 4 cm behind the caudal angle of the scapula and should extend from a point about 10 cm ventral to the dorsal midline to a point approximately 6 to 8 cm from the ventral midline. The conformation of the dog may require some slight modification of these measurements. As a general guide, the fifth intercostal space lies beneath the nipple of the second mammary gland. The first mammary gland is often hard to find; however, the second mammary gland is located at the point of the elbow when the leg is in midflexion. With a #3

76

handle and a #10 blade, the incision should be continued through the first thin layer of muscle (cutaneous trunci). This muscle is so thin that it is often incised with the skin.

When the wound edges are retracted, a sheet of muscle fibers is seen. If it is obscured by fat, it should be carefully dissected away until the muscle is visible. If the incision extends far enough ventrally, careful inspection will reveal two distinct muscle bundles (Fig. 31A). One group of fibers (the latissimus dorsi) runs

Fig. 31. Thoractomy incision. (A) Position of the latissimus dorsi and rectus abdominis muscles. (B) Retraction of the overlying musculature to reveal the scalenus, serratus ventralis, and external intercostal muscles. (C) Retraction of the scalenus muscle and placement of the incision in the external intercostal muscle.

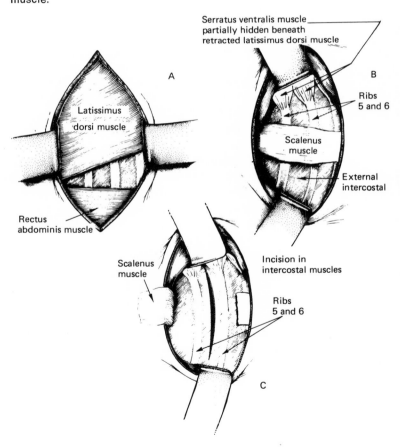

dorsally and caudally, and the other (the rectus abdominis) runs caudally. By careful blunt and sharp dissection, it is possible to separate the fascia jointing these two muscles so that they can be retracted—one dorsally and the other ventrally (Fig. 31B). If the incision is not correctly placed or if the junction of these muscles cannot be found, they can be transected in order to expose the underlying scalenus and intercostal muscles. However, transection can be quite traumatic and result in postoperative complications.

The scalenus muscle fibers transform into its aponeurosis at about the level of the fifth rib. It is quite thin at this point and may be obscured by fat. The aponeurosis of the scalenus muscle is transected, and the muscle is retracted (Fig. 31C).

At this point, the surgeon should make sure that the incision is in the fifth intercostal space by locating the serratus ventralis muscle which extends ventrally to its attachments on the third to the ninth ribs. The first muscle segment is quite small and attaches to the fourth rib. The next two segments are relatively large and attach to the fifth and sixth ribs. These two segments should be carefully separated for the dorsal extension of the incision through the intercostal space.

Two intercostal muscles (external and internal) will be found in each intercostal space. Since the blood supply for these muscles runs along the caudal aspect of each rib, the incision should be placed midway between the fifth and sixth ribs to avoid cutting these vessels. Metzenbaum scissors are used to transect the fibers of the intercostal muscles—first the external and then the internal (the shearing action of instruments like this provides better hemostasis than the blade of a scalpel). At this point the surgeon should inform the anesthetist that he is entering the thoracic cavity, so that positive-pressure ventilation can be started.

The endothoracic fascia and parietal pleura will now emerge as transparent structures, under which the lungs may be seen gliding as they expand and deflate. During expiration, the parietal pleura low in the intercostal space should be punctured with a pair of closed Metzenbaum scissors. The fifth and sixth ribs should then be separated by rib retractors, padded with moist sponges. Be careful not to include any lung tissue between the blades of the retractor and the edge of the incision. From this point on, extreme care must be exercised in handling the thoracic contents. Since air does not clot, gas leaks caused by injury to the lung may result in postoperative pneumothorax and death. For this reason, the lung should not be handled with instruments, but rather with the fingers or with moist sponges.

B. Removing the lobe

The left diaphragmatic lobe should be identified (Fig. 32A) and then pulled gently but firmly cranially in order to expose the left pulmonary ligament (Fig. 32B)—an avascular fold of pleura, which attaches the caudal border of the diaphragmatic lobe to the mediastinal pleura covering the hilus of the lung. Severing this avascular ligament with the Metzenbaum scissors mobilizes the left diaphragmatic lobe so that it can be lifted out of the wound (Fig. 33A). Although the pulmonary ligament is the primary attachment for this lobe, there are usually some other pleural attachments between the diaphragmatic lobe and the mediastinum, especially near the hilus. These other attachments, however, may contain small blood vessels and require careful transection. The fissure separating the diaphragmatic lobe from the cardiac lobe should be bluntly dissected, carefully examining for connective tissue attachments which may contain parenchymal tissue. If present, they should be ligated with 0 silk before transection. By careful dissection, the structures on both the dorsal and the ventral aspect of the hilus are separated from the surrounding connective tissue. These structures, in cranial to caudal order, are the left pulmonary artery, bronchus, and vein (Fig. 33A).

The pulmonary artery should be identified, bluntly dissected from surrounding tissue and triple ligated with 00 silk. Metzenbaum

Fig. 32. Exposing the thoracic contents. (A) After the incision has been made into the thoracic cavity, the ribs are spread with retractors to reveal the underlying thoracic viscera. (B) Craniad retraction of the diaphragmatic lobe exposes the left pulmonary ligament.

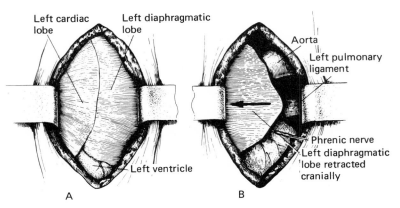

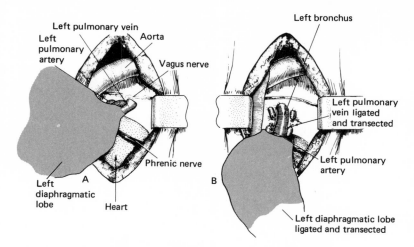

Fig. 33. Hilar attachments of the left diaphragmatic lobe of the lung. (A) The left diaphragmatic lobe has been lifted out of the incision and pulled craniad to allow visualization of the left pulmonary vein as it enters the lobe. (B) Ventral retraction of the diaphragmatic lobe affords visualization of the left pulmonary artery, vein, and bronchus.

scissors should be used to sever the artery between the two most distal ligatures. The pulmonary vein is then ligated and divided in a similar manner (Fig. 33B). The connective tissue in the area should be carefully examined for any additional blood vessels.

The bronchus is double ligated with 00 silk and severed with a pair of Metzenbaum scissors distal to both ligatures. A small flap of pleura is then folded over the stump and oversewn with interrupted sutures of 000 chromic surgical gut. Care should be taken not to place sutures proximal to the ligatures around the bronchus.

C. Inserting a chest tube

Before closing the chest, the surgeon should have a sponge count made and should inspect the operative field to be sure that hemostasis is complete. The thoracic cavity should then be filled with warm (35°–39°C), sterile saline and the bronchial stump observed during inspiration. The occurrence of bubbling indicates an air leak. The remaining lobes should also be inspected for air leaks before aspirating the saline from the thoracic cavity. If air leaks are detected, they must be ligated with 0 silk or umbilical tape. If the leak is large, or multiple, it may be necessary to remove the remaining lung lobes on the left side.

The two methods of aspiration commonly used to reestablish negative pressure in the chest following a thoracotomy are needle puncture and insertion of a chest tube. In this exercise the chest-tube procedure is used and the tube is inserted while the chest is

Fig. 34. Preparation for placement of chest tube. A small skin incision is made 3 to 4 intercostal spaces caudal to the operative site (A), and a curved hemostat is tunneled under the skin to the intercostal space next to the operative site (B). During expiration, the hemostat is thrust through the thoracic wall into the thoracic cavity.

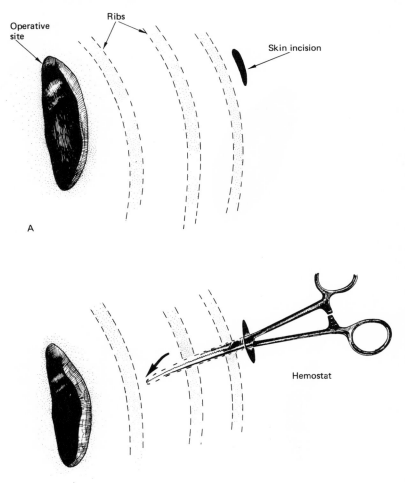

still open. A hemostat is used to pull one end of the tube out through a small skin incision, by the methods shown in Figs. 34 and 35. After the chest is closed, a loose purse-string suture of nonabsorbable suture material is placed in the skin around the tube (Fig. 36C).

Fig. 35. Placement of the chest tube. A tube inserted into the chest through the thoracotomy incision is grasped with the hemostat (A) and pulled under the skin (B) and out through the skin incision, so that only 6–8 cm of tubing remains in the thoracic cavity.

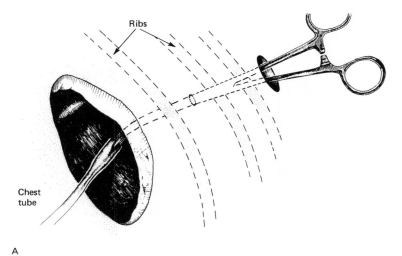

A

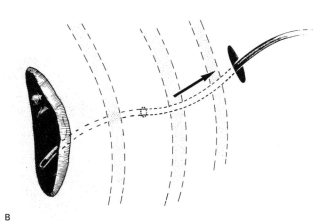

B

D. Closing the incision

In order to close the incision, the fifth and sixth ribs must be approximated. This is done with a minimum of four sutures of 00 stainless steel wire, placed around both ribs by means of a large curved needle with a noncutting edge. When these sutures are being placed, the lungs should be held in expiration by the anesthetist and the assistant surgeon should gently retract them away from the path of the needle. Care must also be taken to avoid the

Fig. 36. Closure of the thoracotomy incision. (A) Apposition of the ribs with preplaced simple interrupted sutures. (B) Reattachment of the aponeurosis of the scalenus muscle. (C) Apposition of the latissimus dorsi and rectus abdominis muscles.

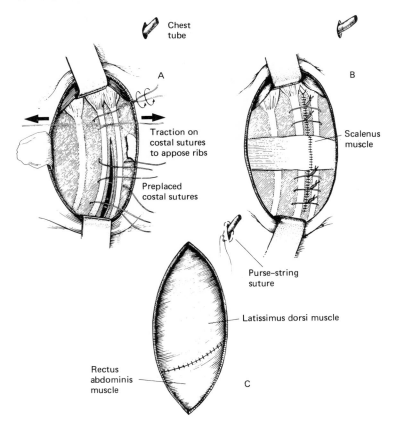

intercostal vessels which lie on the caudal edge of each rib. When the surgeon is ready to tie these preplaced costal sutures, the assistant grasps the ends of the sutures adjacent to the sutures to be tied and pulls them in opposite directions (Fig. 36A). This will hold the ribs together while the surgeon ties the adjacent suture ends. The sutures should be twisted together six to eight times, rather than tying in a square knot, to maintain proximation for subsequent suturing of the soft tissue. This procedure should start at one end of the incision and continue until all are tied. The ribs, at this point, should just be in apposition; too much tension will cause them to override each other and interfere with closure of the soft tissues.

The intercostal muscles should be sutured with simple interrupted sutures of 00 chromic surgical gut (Fig. 36B). A small amount of sterile saline should be dropped along the incision line to test it for air leaks. If there are any leaks, loose fascia is sutured in place over the incision site with simple interrupted sutures of 00 chromic surgical gut.

The transected aponeurosis of the scalenus muscle can be sutured with simple interrupted sutures of 00 chromic surgical gut (Fig. 36B). The ventral edge of the latissimus dorsi muscle may be reattached to the dorsal edge of the rectus abdominis muscle with a simple continuous suture of 00 chromic surgical gut (Fig. 36C).

To eliminate dead space, the subcutaneous tissues should be reunited by a simple continuous suture of 00 chromic surgical gut. Finally, the skin is closed with simple interrupted sutures of nonabsorbable suture material on a cutting-edge needle.

E. Reestablishing respiration

After a three-way stopcock has been attached to the chest tube, the lungs are inflated. At the peak of inspiration, the chest tube is clamped with a hemostat and a 50-ml syringe is attached to the stopcock. The hemostat is released while air and/or fluid are aspirated from the chest cavity through the syringe. The surgeon reclamps the chest tube, and positive-pressure ventilation is stopped. If the dog does not start breathing in 2 or 3 minutes, positive-pressure ventilation should be given intermittently until voluntary respiration is observed. The chest tube should be aspirated every 15 minutes for the first hour, and hourly thereafter until three consecutive aspirations each yield less than 10 ml of air of fluid. The chest tube may then be removed and the purse-string suture pulled taut.

III. Postsurgical Care

In addition to the routine postsurgical care described in Chapter 6, the dog's respiratory pattern should be carefully checked and his chest auscultated at least once a day for 3 days following the operation. The color of the mucous membranes and the capillary-refilling time should also be checked at least twice daily.

On postsurgical day 1, a blood sample is collected from the femoral artery for determination of the pH, p_{CO_2}, and p_{O_2}.

IV. Clinical Considerations

In order to analyze the results of this procedure and to understand the complex physiological alterations which have taken place, the student should review the discussions of these mechanisms in the texts by Comroe, 1965; Guyton, 1966; and Soma, 1971.

The left diaphragmatic lobe of the lung represents approximately one fourth of the dog's total lung capacity. When this lobe is removed, those portions of the blood and of the inhaled gases normally coming to that lobe for gaseous exchange are rerouted, by vascular and gaseous shunting mechanisms, to reserve areas in other portions of the lung. The net result of these processes is a normal blood pH, p_{CO_2} and p_{O_2} but a decreased respiratory reserve. This reduction in reserve capacity may become clinically apparent as a decreased tolerance for exercise.

9

Ligation of a Coronary Artery

C. MAX LANG AND HOWARD C. HUGHES

The occlusion of a coronary artery, whether by surgery or by an obstruction, normally causes ischemia in the portion of myocardium supplied by that artery. The degree of ischemia and the resultant interruption of function are related to the level at which the coronary artery is occluded.

I. Coronary Circulation

A. Anatomy

In dogs, the heart normally lies between the walls of the mediastinal pleura and extends from the level of the third rib to the inferior border of the sixth rib.

The right coronary artery arises from the right coronary sinus of the aorta (Fig. 37A). It encircles the right side of the heart in the coronary sulcus; however, it rarely crosses the crux heart as it normally does in man. The right coronary artery provides blood to the bulk of the right atrium and ventricle, except in the areas immediately adjacent to the interventricular septum.

The left main coronary artery is about twice as large as the right and arises from the base of the aorta in the left coronary sinus. It supplies blood to the left ventricle, left atrium, entire septum, and a portion of the right ventricle adjacent to the interventricular sulci. The left coronary artery is only a few millimeters in length and

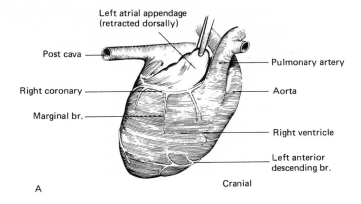

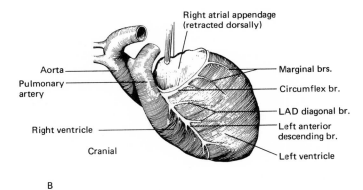

Fig. 37. Lateral surfaces of the canine heart; (A) right and (B) left.

divides into the left anterior descending (LAD) and the circumflex coronary artery (Fig. 37B).

The LAD comes around the pulmonary artery and emerges from under the tip of the atrial appendage after its first diagonal branch. It continues down the interventricular sulci on the sternal surface of the heart, giving off 3–4 other major diagonal branches. These diagonal vessels supply the ventrolateral aspect of the left ventricle.

The circumflex coronary artery goes caudally around the heart in the atrioventricular sulcus (usually covered with fat and located at the edge of the left atrial appendage) before it emerges on the caudal surface of the heart as the posterior descending coronary artery. The marginal branches of the circumflex coronary artery supply the lateral wall of the left ventricle. The coronary veins of the dog, unlike man, usually occur in pairs and accompany each coronary artery, one on each side.

B. Physiology

The heart beats because of a stimulus (impulse, wave of depolarization, wave of electrical negativity) which originates within the heart at the sinoatrial node, located near the junction of the anterior vena cava with the right atrium. Because of the syncytial nature of cardiac muscle, stimulation of any single atrial or ventricular muscle fiber causes the action potential to travel over the entire muscle mass of the atrium or ventricle. If the atrioventricular (AV) bundle is intact, the action potential passes from the atria to the ventricles.

The intensity and direction of these electrical stimuli as they travel through the cardiac muscle can be measured by the electrocardiograph. Many abnormalities of the cardiac muscle can be detected by analyzing the contours of the waves in the different electrocardiographic leads.

In order to contract, the myocardium must have an adequate supply of chemical energy. This energy is derived mainly from the oxidative metabolism of fatty acids and, to a lesser extent, of glucose and other nutrients. Any interruption in the supply of fatty acids and oxygen, or decreased removal of metabolites, can seriously affect the ability of the heart to function.

II. Surgical Procedure

To demonstrate the effects of varying degrees of occlusion, different surgical teams can ligate the LAD, circumflex coronary, or right coronary artery at different levels. The LAD and circumflex coronary artery ligation is done through a thoracotomy on the left side and the right coronary artery ligation is done through one on the right side.

The thoracotomy incision for this procedure is the same as that described for the lobectomy (Chapter 8). The initial incision through the pleura is made by a small nick, and a grooved director is then inserted beneath the pleura to protect the lung. The pleura is usually incised simultaneously with the intercostal muscles. The anesthetist must begin positive-pressure ventilation as soon as the thoracic cavity is entered, but he should be asked to stop lung inflation momentarily while the pleural incision is completed. Saline moistened sponges are placed on the cut surface of the intercostal muscles to prevent drying. Rib retractors are then inserted and expanded (while the lungs are held in expiration) to expose the operative field. Pack the lungs caudally with saline moistened sponges to expose the heart in its pericardial sac. Periodically (every 10 to 15 minutes) throughout the procedure, the anesthetist should hyperinflate the lungs to correct atelectasis.

The pericardium is incised perpendicular to the phrenic nerve by picking it up with smooth thumb forceps, nicking it with the scalpel, and extending the incision with Metzenbaum scissors. The incision is started about 0.5–1 cm ventral to the phrenic nerve and is extended to the apex of the heart. The heart is then gently removed from its pericardial sac for better exposure.

To visualize the left coronary artery, the surgeon should gently lift the atrial appendage and retract the pulmonary artery. The origins of the LAD and circumflex coronary arteries may not be readily visible because they are usually buried in fat. However, the LAD artery can usually be seen as it emerges from the fat in the atrioventricular sulcus. The visibility of the circumflex coronary artery may vary, since it often dips in and out of this fat. The marginal vessels, however, are quite distinct as they emerge from this fat perpendicular to the atrioventricular sulcus.

The right coronary artery lies under the atrial appendage; and it, too, is often covered by fat. It is usually visible several centimeters distal to its emergence from under the appendage.

The surgeon should, as gently as possible, bluntly dissect the vessel to be ligated from any surrounding fat. If either the artery or one of its accompanying veins is accidentally torn, ligate the vessel above and below the site with 00 silk on a curved atraumatic needle. If the artery is successfully dissected free, only one ligation in the same manner is necessary.

The high LAD artery ligation should be placed as it emerges from beneath the atrial appendage and below the first diagonal branch (if the ligature is placed too high on either coronary artery, it can result in fibrillation and death). If the LAD artery is to be ligated low, it should be done just below the origin of the second or third diagonal branch.

The high circumflex coronary artery ligation should be placed just proximal to the origin of the first major marginal branch and the low ligation just distal to it.

Before the pericardium is closed (with a continuous suture of

00 silk), the surgeon should watch the ischemia developing in the myocardium. This is the initial stage of a myocardial infarct, and is rarely observed.

The pericardium is closed with a simple continuous pattern using 00 silk. Closure of the thoracotomy is the same as described for the lobectomy (Chapter 8). The insertion of a chest tube is normally used to reestablish negative pressure in the chest. However, an alternative method is needle aspiration using a sterile 50-ml syringe equipped with a three-way valve and a 16-gauge needle. The needle should be inserted above the dorsal border of the lungs in the ninth or tenth intercostal space. Care must be taken not to penetrate the lung with the needle during insertion or the process of aspiration. Aspiration should be done until negative pressure is reestablished.

III. Postsurgical Care

Basic postsurgical care is the same as that previously described in Chapter 6.

An electrocardiogram should be taken preoperatively and on postsurgical days 1, 7, and 14. Leads to be recorded are I, II, III, aVR, aVL, and aVF. At the same time, blood samples are collected for the following determinations: White cell and differential counts; serum creatinine phosphokinase (CPK); lactic acid dehydrogenase (LDH), total and isoenzymes; and α-hydroxybutyrate dehydrogenase (HBD).

IV. Cardiac Resuscitation

Ligation of any coronary artery produces an area of ischemia in the myocardium. This ischemic area can initiate an electrical signal, resulting in premature ventricular contractions. This is reflected on the electrocardiogram as a widened Q wave and bizarre QRS complex, occurring early and not preceded by a P wave. It is typically followed by a compensatory pause, i.e., isoelectric activity. If severe, the animal may develop ventricular fibrillation. This type of arrythmia is reflected on the electrocardiogram as undulating, bizarre baseline movements, without any evidence of atrial activity or of T waves. This can, of course, result in death if immediate corrective action is not taken.

The goal of treatments for acute cardiac failure is to (1) restore and maintain blood flow to the vital organs, and (2) to reinitiate normal cardiac contractions.

In the case of an acute cardiac failure, one should start cardiac massage immediately to maintain blood flow to the vital organs. If the thoracic cavity is open, this can be done by grasping the heart in the palm of the hand and rhythmically squeezing it at a rate of 70 times per minute. If the thoracic cavity is closed, cardiac massage is done by compressing the dog's chest on the left side with the palm of the hand over the heart at the level of the costal cartilage.

An open airway must be established and maintained during cardiac massage. The animal should be intubated and positive pressure given at the rate of 20 respirations per minute. If artificial respiration and external cardiac massage are required simultaneously, the chest should be compressed 6 to 7 times for each respiration.

A defibrillator can be used to correct fibrillation. To reestablish normal conduction, the defibrillator places a direct electrical current across the heart, producing complete depolarization of the cardiac muscle. The current is transmitted from the device to the heart by means of "paddles." The paddles should be moistened with sterile saline for open-chest defibrillation, and electrocardiographic paste for closed-chest defibrillation to ensure good electrical contact.

Approximately 10 to 50 W-seconds of power are used for open-chest defibrillation and 50 to 500 W-seconds for closed-chest defibrillation. One should start with the lower setting and gradually increase it to minimize "burning" of the heart. Prior to the defibrillator discharge, all personnel should stand away from the patient to avoid injury.

If the defibrillation cannot be corrected after three attempts, and the thoracic cavity is open, remove the coronary artery ligature. Then massage the heart until the ischemic area is reperfused with blood and attempt defibrillation again.

Drug therapy is also used in conjunction with these procedures. Lidocaine, 50 mg i.v., can be used to stabilize the membrane potentials. Acidosis can be prevented, or reversed, with sodium bicarbonate (20 mEq i.v.). If the equipment is available, blood gases should be determined for the acid–base status. If there is acidosis, the sodium bicarbonate is given at a rate of 3 mEq for each increment of deficit.

Epinephrine (1 ml of a 1:10,000 solution) can be given i.v. (or intracardiac for an immediate response) to improve the heart rate and strength of contraction. Calcium chloride or calcium gluconate can also be given (200 to 300 mg i.v.) to improve the strength of contraction.

Isoproterenol is used to increase peripheral venous constriction and, as a result, increase the amount of blood returning to the heart. However, since it is a very potent beta-adrenergic stimulator, it must be diluted prior to administration. One milliliter of a 1:5000 solution of isoproterenol is diluted in 100 ml of 5% dextrose in saline and given i.v. at the rate of 1 to 2 ml/minute.

V. Clinical Considerations

A. Pathophysiology and myocardial infarction

Acute myocardial infarction is a clinical syndrome that results from a sudden and persistent interruption of the blood supply to a part of the myocardium. The occurrence and extent of infarction depend primarily on the site of infarction and on the distribution of blood supply from the various branches of the coronary arteries. The former determines the amount of collateral circulation available from proximal branches of the affected artery and from neighboring arteries.

In some cases it is possible for the collateral circulation to maintain viability of the myocardium in spite of an infarction. Even in these cases, however, blood flow from the coronary arteries to the myocardium is usually insufficient to prevent ischemia. Because metabolism of the muscle is depressed by (1) oxygen deficit; (2) excess metabolite accumulation such as carbon dioxide, lactate, potassium, and ADP; and (3) lack of sufficient nutrients, depolarization of the membranes cannot occur in areas of severe myocardial ischemia; consequently, the function of the heart can be severely impaired even though the myocardium does not die.

B. Myocardial infarction in man

An acute myocardial infarction is characterized by severe and prolonged cardiac pain, fever, leukocytosis, and electrocardiographic and laboratory evidence of myocardial necrosis. The elevation of temperature is slight, usually beginning after the infarction and returning to normal within a week. Leukocytosis occurs regularly, often within a few hours, and disappears before the end of a week if there are no complications.

The myocardium contains large quantities of certain enzymes—notably CPK, LDH and HBD. Increased concentrations of these enzymes are found in the blood after a myocardial infarct and can be used as a rough index to the extent of myocardial necrosis.

LDH is found in organs other than the heart, but the concentration of its five components (isoenzymes) varies in different organs. The concentration of these isoenzymes in the peripheral blood can be determined by a combination of spectrophotometric and electrophoretic techniques. Isoenzymes 1 and 2 are present predominantly in the myocardium, and their activity in the serum is increased for periods of 1 to 3 weeks following myocardial necrosis.

The HBD activity in the serum corresponds to LDH 1 and 2 activity. Serum levels of HBD remain elevated for 7 to 10 days following myocardial damage.

CPK is more specific for acute myocardial infarction than LDH, since it is found in very high concentrations in the myocardium. Its early elevation (within 6 hours after the infarct) is another advantage.

Electrocardiographic changes are usually found within the first 24 hours after an acute infarction, and sometimes within the first few hours. They occasionally persist for more than 24 hours but are relatively uncommon after the first 10 days. The electrocardiographic changes usually suggest the location of the infarct (transmural, subendocardial, on the diaphragmatic wall, etc.).

These changes generally consist of abnormal Q waves, elevation of the S–T segment and, less frequently, depression of the S–T segment and T wave changes. The Q waves are prolonged and deeper than usual, indicating a loss of potential in the muscle. Elevation of the S–T segments denotes subepicardial injury. Inversion of the T wave indicates ischemia of the myocardium in areas adjacent to the necrotic tissue, and a disturbance in repolarization of the affected ventricle.

C. Myocardial infarction in the dog

In the dog, however, these changes are transitory and are not usually detected by ordinary electrocardiographic means. The major changes seen in the dog consist primarily of premature ventricular contraction, which usually only occurs with the high ligations. Premature ventricular contractions can be dangerous in that if one should occur during the vulnerable period of the cardiac cycle (T wave) ventricular fibrillation can occur. One should attempt to prevent these premature contractions especially if the occurrence is greater than three consecutively. Membrane stabilizing agents such as lidocaine (50 mg given rapid i.v.) will usually abolish the premature contractions. Additional lidocaine may be used, however, the total dose should not exceed 4 mg/kg within a 2-hour period since overdose can produce asystole.

10

Nephrectomy

HOWARD C. HUGHES, WM. J. WHITE,
AND C. MAX LANG

Nephrectomy (Gk. *nephros,* kidney and Gr. *ektomē,* excision) is defined as "excision of a kidney."[1] This surgical procedure, alone or in combination with other related procedures, can be used to study several biological phenomena. These include (1) nephrectomy—mechanism of renal compensation by the remaining kidney; (2) nephrectomy, followed by the application of a Goldblatt clamp to the artery supplying the remaining kidney—development of renal hypertension; and (3) transplanting the excised kidney—transplantation biology.

I. Kidneys

A. Anatomy

The canine kidneys are dark-brown organs, shaped like plump beans and imbedded in adipose capsules. They are located retroperitoneally in the lumbar region—one on each side of the vertebral column (Fig. 38). The right kidney lies at the level of the first three lumbar vertebrae; the left kidney, at the level of the second, third, and fourth lumbar vertebrae. The close proximity of the right kidney to the inferior vena cava necessitates extreme care in resecting it. The superior aspect of the left kidney is in

---

[1] Dorland's *Illustrated Medical Dictionary* (1974). 25th ed. Philadelphia: W. B. Saunders Co.

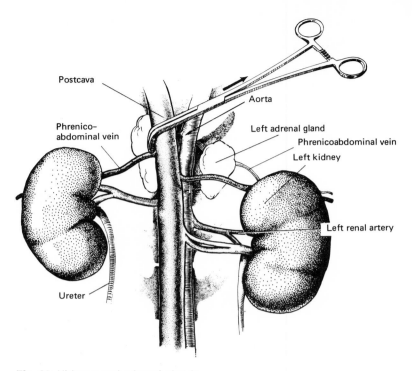

Fig. 38. Kidneys and adrenal glands.

contact with the medial surface of the spleen, the greater omentum, and the greater curvature of the stomach. The adrenal glands are located just above the superior pole of each kidney.

In most dogs, the renal artery divides into two branches just before it enters the hilus of the kidney (Fig. 38); more rarely, two separate arteries pass directly from the aorta to the hilus. Normally, blood from each kidney drains into one vein passing from the hilus to the inferior vena cava; occasionally, however, there are veins emptying into the vena cava from other areas of the kidney.

B. Physiology

The kidney has two major functions: (1) the excretion of waste products from catabolism, and (2) the regulation of homeostasis through acid–base balance and osmolarity. Although acid–base balance is primarily controlled by the lungs, the kidneys play a major role in conserving bicarbonate and eliminating nonvolatile acids. Hence, the kidney is the organ ultimately responsible for maintaining acid–base balance. Osmolarity is regulated by the excretion and resorption of electrolytes and water.

Because of the kidneys' important role in maintaining homeostasis, blood flow to these organs is closely regulated by the renin–angiotensin–aldosterone mechanism for controlling blood pressure. When blood flow to the kidneys decreases, renin is released from the juxtaglomerular apparatus. Renin converts angiotensin (from the liver) to angiotensin I, which, in turn, is converted into angiotensin II. Angiotensin II, besides being a very potent vasopressor, stimulates the release of aldosterone from the adrenal gland. Aldosterone also has some vasopressor activity, although its principal function is to increase the resorption of sodium and the excretion of potassium.

II. Surgical Procedure

A. Nephrectomy

Depending primarily on the surgeon's preference, nephrectomy may be done either through an incision in the flank region or through a midline abdominal incision. However, the former is more difficult.

1. *Flank incision technique*

The skin incision, made with a #20 blade in a #4 handle, begins at the paralumbar fossa, approximately 3 cm caudal to the last rib, and extends ventrocaudally at a 45° angle (Fig. 39). If this approach is employed, three muscle layers will be incised: external oblique, internal oblique, and transverse abdominal. The direction of the muscle fibers in these three layers is, respectively, caudoventral, cranioventral, and dorsoventral. After the fascia of each muscle layer has been cut with a #10 blade in a #3 handle, the muscle tissue is bluntly dissected along the line of its fibers. The surgeon must be careful not to sever the iliohypogastric nerve, which arises from the ventral root of the first three lumbar nerves and runs ventrally between the external and the internal oblique muscles in the area of this incision.

The flank incision technique permits the surgeon to remove the kidney retroperitoneally without entering the abdominal cavity. Because the peritoneum is attached to the transverse abdominal muscle, however, it is often incised accidentally when the muscle fibers are separated.

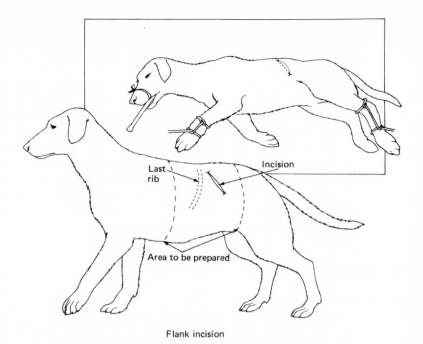

Flank incision

Fig. 39. Site of the flank incision for nephrectomy. The insert shows a dog in the right lateral recumbent position.

2. *Midline incision technique*

This is the laparotomy incision described in Chapter 6. To assure sufficient space for manipulation within the abdominal cavity, the incision should extend from a point 3 cm distal to the xiphoid cartilage to a point 4 cm distal to the umbilicus.

The intestines are packed with a sterile laparotomy sponge moistened in saline. Picking up the peritoneum at one pole of the kidney with a pair of forceps to make a tent, the surgeon nicks it with the Metzenbaum scissors and, by means of blunt dissection, carefully separates the peritoneum from the surface of the kidney and its vessels.

3. *Removing the kidney*

While the flank or midline incision is held open with a Balfour retractor, the surgeon uses his finger to separate the kidney from its surrounding fat pad by blunt dissection. He then gently lifts the kidney to expose the dorsal surface of the hilus. First the renal artery and then the vein are carefully dissected along their length and ligated, each with three separate ligatures of 00 silk. If the kidney appears to enlarge and become turgid after the vein is tied off, an additional arterial supply should be sought and immediately ligated.

After the vessels are cut between the two ligatures closest to the kidney, the organ is carefully inspected for any aberrant vessels and then lifted out of the incision. The ureter is ligated in two places with 00 silk and severed between the two ligatures.

After all sponges and instruments have been removed, the surgeon carefully checks the area for bleeding. The incision is closed in the manner previously described (Chapter 6).

B. Placing the goldblatt clamp

If the midline incision technique was used, the Goldblatt clamp can be applied before the peritoneum is closed. It is preferable, however, to wait until a later date (at least 2 weeks), after the remaining kidney has compensated. If the clamp is applied at the time of nephrectomy, saline-moistened sterile laparotomy sponges are used to pack the intestines away from the remaining kidney. After carefully dissecting the peritoneum, connective tissue, and fat from the renal artery, the Goldblatt clamp (Fig. 40) is placed on the artery so that the top and bottom plates just touch the opposite surfaces of the vessel. The clamp is then removed and the number of turns needed to close the plates completely are

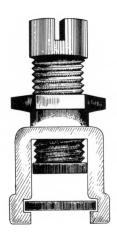

Fig. 40. Goldblatt clamp.

|← 5 mm →|

counted. Once again, the clamp is placed on the renal artery so that the top and bottom plates just touch the opposite surfaces. By counting the number of turns, the distance between the plates is reduced to occlude the vessel by approximately one third.

If the renal artery is occluded to the point that blood flow through the kidney is inadequate for normal excretory function, uremia[2] will develop and the animal will die. If, on the other hand, the renal artery is insufficiently occluded, hypertension will not develop.

Excessive handling of the renal artery must be avoided, since additional occlusion of the vessel by intravascular edema can also cause uremia and death. If there are two renal arteries, the diameter of the larger one is measured by application of the clamp before the smaller artery is ligated, and the clamp is then reapplied as described previously. Unless this sequence is followed, the expansion of the artery that follows ligation of the secondary blood supply would make it difficult to judge the correct amount of occlusion.

Before closing the abdomen, the surgeon should palpate the renal artery distal to the Goldblatt clamp for pulsations and check the color and texture of the kidney to verify that an adequate blood supply is available for normal excretory function. After all sponges and packing have been removed, the area is again carefully inspected for bleeding. The intestines are replaced in their normal position, and the incision is closed in the manner described in Chapter 6.

C. Renal transplant

This procedure involves two surgical sites: the abdomen for removal of the kidney to be transplanted and the neck as the recipient site. The recipient site is prepared first. Make a ventral midline skin incision, with a #20 blade in a #4 handle, from the hyoid bone of the larynx to the manubrium junction. Bluntly dissect the fascia between the sternohyoideus muscles to expose the trachea. Be very careful not to enter the thoracic cavity at the thoracic inlet. Locate the carotid artery and the vagal and sympathetic nerve trunks which lie in a sheath approximately 2 cm dorsolateral to the trachea. Palpation of the carotid artery pulse will help to locate this sheath. Isolate the artery by blunt dissection

---

[2] The chief biochemical sign of uremia is severe azotemia. The total clinical picture includes malnutrition, anemia, acidosis, water and electrolyte imbalance, severe hypertensive vascular disease, and circulatory insufficiency.

for approximately 6 cm along its length and carefully remove all adventitia. This is very important because any remaining adventitia will interfere with subsequent suturing of the vessels. The external jugular vein lies subcutaneously, approximately 4 cm from the midline, over the sternocephalicus muscle. Isolate the vein and remove its adventitia. After this is completed cover the area with sterile sponges moistened with saline and proceed with the abdominal incision.

The abdominal incision is the same as that previously described for the nephrectomy. After the peritoneum has been removed from over the kidney, being careful not to remove the renal capsule, isolate the renal vessels of the left kidney from the hilus to the aorta and inferior vena cava. Clamp the renal artery near its origin from the aorta with a hemostat. Inject 10 ml of heparinized saline with a 25-gauge needle into the artery distal to the clamp to prevent coagulation of the blood in the kidney. Clamp the renal vein with a hemostat near the inferior vena cava. Double ligate the renal artery and vein, separately, proximal to the clamp with 00 silk and cut the vessels distal to the clamp. Remove the clamps from the renal artery and vein. Bluntly dissect the perirenal fat from the kidney and ureter. Double ligate the ureter approximately 4 cm proximal to its insertion into the urinary bladder and cut proximal to the two ligatures. Place the kidney in a pan of cold (4°C) heparinized saline and remove the adventitia from the renal vessels. The abdomen is temporarily closed with warm moist towels.

The next step is to return to the recipient site in the neck. Clamp the carotid artery and jugular vein individually as close to the thoracic inlet as possible with bulldog clamps. Double ligate these vessels as far cephalad as possible and cut just proximal to the ligatures. Flush the blood out of the vessels with heparinized saline. There should be at least 3 cm between the bulldog clamp and the cut end. Remove any remaining adventitia from the vessel ends for at least 1 cm. Bring the carotid artery out from under the sternocephalicus so that it lies alongside the jugular vein.

Place the kidney in the implant site and position it for anastomosis. The vessels will be sutured using 4–0 synthetic nonabsorbable material. A triangulation suture pattern is used for the anastomosis. The two ends of the vessels are brought into apposition using three separate stay sutures placed 120° apart on the circumference of the vessel (Fig. 41A). The suture placement should be about 1 mm from the cut ends of the vessel. Tie each stay suture with at least 5 knots, but do not cut the ends. The assistant should then pick

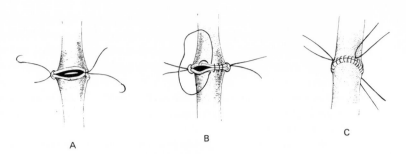

Fig. 41. Vascular anastomosis using a triangulation suture pattern. Stay sutures are placed (A); the ends of the vessels are sutured with a continuous suture pattern (B); and (C) the suture ends are tied and cut.

up the loose ends (without needles) of two adjacent stay sutures and hold them so the suture line is straight and visible to the surgeon. The surgeon then sutures from one stay suture to the other, using a simple continuous pattern (Fig. 41B). Each suture should be 1 mm apart.

Tie the needle end of the first stay suture to the loose end of the second stay suture. The assistant should then pick up the loose ends of the second and third stay sutures, and rotate the field of view to the surgeon. The surgeon proceeds toward the third, using the needle end of the second stay suture. Repeat again from the third to the first stay suture. Cut all ends after all of the sutures have been tied (Fig. 41C).

The arteries should be anastomosed first and then the veins. Care must be taken to prevent twisting and subsequent occlusion of the vessels.

When all of the anastomoses are completed, release the bulldog clamp from the jugular vein. Retrograde filling will permit visualization of any leaks. Place a simple interrupted suture at any site on the anastomosis which continues to bleed for more than 3 minutes. Release the clamp from the carotid artery, and again observe for leakage. In addition, observe the kidney for color as well as urine production. The kidney can survive for approximately 1 hour after its blood supply is removed without residual damage. Therefore, it is important to complete the vascular anastomoses in as short a period of time as possible.

Prepare a subcutaneous bed in the loose connective tissue of the ventrolateral neck area and place the kidney in it without twisting or occluding the vessels. Make a stab wound in the skin over the hilus of the kidney and pull the ureter through with mosquito forceps. Catheterize the ureter with polyethelene tubing, then suture it to the skin using a simple interrupted pattern with 4–0 silk suture.

Close the dead space of the pocket in which the kidney lies with 0 medium chromic surgical gut. Close the skin with nonabsorbable suture material using a horizontal mattress suture pattern. The ureter should be closely observed for urine production. If no urine is produced, reexamine the kidney and the vascular anastomoses. If the kidney is swollen and dark blue, carefully examine the vein for twisting or occlusion. If the kidney is soft and pale, examine the artery for patency. Corrective action must be taken at once or the kidney will be rejected.

III. Postsurgical Care

A. Nephrectomy

Basic postsurgical care is the same as that previously described (Chapter 6). Blood and urine samples should be collected on days 1, 3, 5, and 7 postoperatively and submitted to the laboratory for the following determinations:

1. Urine pH and specific gravity
2. Blood urea nitrogen
3. Serum creatinine
4. Serum sodium, potassium, and chloride

In addition, daily observations should be made and recorded on urine volume and frequency of urination. These laboratory data should be compared with preoperative values to assess the effects of the surgical procedure.

B. Goldblatt clamp

If the Goldblatt clamp procedure was done, at the time of the nephrectomy or later, the dog's blood pressure should also be taken on days 1, 3, 5, and 7. The use of the sphygmomanometer to measure the blood pressure in the dog is described in Chapter 17. The laboratory determinations and blood pressure measurements should also be repeated on day 14. Hypertension, as a result of this surgical procedure, should be detected within 7–10 days using these determinations.

C. Renal transplant

The basic postsurgical care for the nephrectomy procedure is also followed for the renal transplant. The neck area should be kept clean to prevent "urine burns."

The function of the transplanted kidney should be evaluated using specific tests. Starting on postsurgical day 2, collect three consecutive 20-minute samples of urine from the transplanted kidney. Inject 20% mannitol solution (2 ml/kg of body weight) and repeat the three consecutive 20-minute urine samples. Measure the volume, pH, and specific gravity of all samples. This should be repeated on postoperative day 4 with hydrochlorothiazide (10 ml/kg body weight) intramuscularly, and on day 6 with aqueous vasopressin (5 mu/kg body weight) i.v.

IV. Clinical Considerations

The removal of a kidney is usually followed by a compensatory hypertrophy of the remaining one. Although the exact mechanism for this is unknown, it is believed to have some neurologic involvement. The compensation is relatively rapid and not usually detected by changes in the blood or urine.

A. Renal hypertension

Hypertension and renal pathology are often interrelated, and either can predispose to the other. Anything that significantly decreases renal function usually produces hypertension. Although the exact mechanism of renal hypertension has not yet been proven, there are two principal theories:

1. *The renin–angiotensin theory.* Some investigators believe that an excess of renin is excreted by the kidney under certain abnormal conditions. The resultant arteriolar constriction and increase in aldosterone lead to the retention of fluids and electrolytes in the body.
2. *The increased extracellular-fluid volume theory.* This is based on the direct relationship between reduced kidney function and retention of increasing amounts of extracellular fluid.

Hypertension in man can result from unilateral renal pathology, and correction of the predisposing cause can result in a return to the normotensive state. In the dog, however, unilateral renal pathology will not normally cause hypertension. To produce hypertension based on renal ischemia, it is necessary to remove one kidney and reduce the blood flow to the other by means of the Goldblatt clamp.

If the Goldblatt clamp is correctly applied, a syndrome resembling malignant hypertension will result. Blood pressure is increased by 50–100%, and after a few weeks the elevated pressure causes acute fibrinoid degeneration in the arterioles of the kidney, pancreas, mesentery, adrenals, and retina. In the kidney, the acute narrowing of the arteriolar lumen causes diminution of function, with resultant proteinuria and, eventually, chronic renal failure.

Although functional patterns and clinical manifestations can vary early in the course of chronic renal disease, they all tend to become similar as renal failure progresses. Potassium metabolism is usually normal until relatively late in the course of chronic renal insufficiency; then the reduced renal clearance leads to hyperkalemia. Although sodium depletion (hyponatremia) is common in patients with malignant hypertension, it is usually the result of vomiting, diarrhea, or restriction of the sodium intake. Chronic renal failure alone usually decreases the ability of the kidney to vary sodium excretion in either direction. Severe renal failure is usually characterized by an increase in blood urea nitrogen and creatinine.

If the Goldblatt clamp is removed, renal blood flow returns to normal and the signs and symptoms of hypertension and chronic renal failure usually disappear, unless irreversible changes have been produced.

B. Transplantation biology

The transplantation of a single normal kidney in a patient with advanced renal failure (along with the removal of the diseased kidneys) is capable of restoring him to good health for as long as the transplanted kidney continues to function normally. This is a relatively new approach in the treatment of chronic renal diseases but is still in the developmental stage. Although the technical problems of the surgery have been solved, the major problem is that of immunologic rejection.

Rejection does not occur in isologous grafts (i.e., identical twins) because the genetic constitutions of the donor and recipient are the same and, as a result, the tissue antigens are identical. Isologous renal transplants usually function well although there have been some technical failures and, in a few instances, the transplanted kidney appeared to develop the same disease to which the patient's own kidneys succumbed.

When the donor and recipient are of different genetic constitutions, regardless if the same (homograft) or different (heterograft) species, transplantation initiates a complex immune reaction between the host and the graft. This immune response can eventually destroy the graft. Homografts between closely related individuals usually cause mild rejection reactions that can normally be suppressed (at least temporarily) by the use of adrenal steroids and immunosuppressive drugs.

11

Adrenalectomy

WILLIAM J. WHITE AND C. MAX LANG

Adrenalectomy (L. *ad,* near; L. *ren,* kidney; and Gk. *ektomē,* excision) is the term used to denote the surgical removal of one or both adrenal glands.[1] Removal of both of these glands causes severe physiologic changes which are often difficult to correct with replacement therapy. In clinical practice, therefore, bilateral adrenalectomy is rarely used except in cases of adrenal neoplasia.

Removal of the adrenal glands from a dog will give the student surgeon experience in endocrine surgery and in the subsequent use of replacement therapy to maintain homeostasis.

I. Adrenal Glands

A. Anatomy

The canine adrenal glands are flattened, bilobed organs located cranial and medial to the kidneys on either side of the vertebral column (Fig. 38). Each gland is composed of a cortex and a medulla, which are developmentally and functionally separate.

The right adrenal gland, like the right kidney, is situated higher than the corresponding organ on the left. The adrenal glands are bordered cranially by the crura of the diaphragm, and laterally by the cranial poles of the kidneys. The medial surface of the right

---

[1] Dorland's *Illustrated Medical Dictionary* (1974). 25th ed. Philadelphia: W. B. Saunders Co.

adrenal borders on the postcava; however, the entire gland is often hidden by this vein. The left adrenal gland is separated by a small amount of fat and connective tissue from the aorta and postcava. The ventral surface of each adrenal gland is covered by peritoneum; the caudal border is often covered by perirenal fat as well.

The adrenal glands are well supplied with nerves and blood vessels; however, the size of these structures is so small that they are of little significance in this surgical procedure. The middle, cranial, and caudal adrenal arteries normally arise from the aorta, the phrenic artery, and the renal artery; the accessory phrenic and lumbar arteries and occasionally the cranial mesenteric or celiac artery also give off branches to the adrenal glands. Most of the blood leaving each adrenal gland drains into a single adrenal vein. The right adrenal vein empties into the postcava, and the left into the renal vein.

The nerve supply to the adrenal glands comes mainly from the splanchnic nerves, but fibers from the celiac ganglion and from the first three or four ganglia of the abdominal sympathetic chain also innervate these glands.

B. Physiology

The adrenal *medulla* secretes catecholamines (epinephrine and norephinephrine); the cortex secretes a number of steroid hormones, including glucocorticoids, mineralocorticoids, and sex hormones.

The *catecholamines* secreted by the adrenal medulla are probably not essential for life, but they are very valuable in helping to overcome stress. In the dog and in man, epinephrine makes up 80% of the adrenal catecholamine output. Since both norepinephrine and epinephrine are rapidly catabolized in the peripheral circulation, their actions are short-lived. In addition to their metabolic effects (which include gluconeogenesis, mobilization of free fatty acids, and stimulation of the metabolic rate), both of these catecholamines have vaso- and cardioactive properties. They are released from the adrenal medulla mainly by nervous stimulation.

Of the various *glucocorticoids* released by the adrenal cortex, cortisol (hydrocortisone) is the most abundant. The metabolic effects of glucocorticoids are quite varied. They stimulate gluconeogenesis and increase liver glycogen and the concentration of glucose and amino acids in the blood. Glucocorticoids also decrease the cellular utilization of glucose, increase the mobilization of free fatty acids, and make the blood vessels more responsive to the action of catecholamines. The *absence* of glucocorticoids results in abnormal water, carbohydrate, protein, and fat metabolism which may lead to collapse and death following exposure to stress.

Mineralocorticoids, which are also produced in the adrenal cortex, increase the reabsorption of sodium from the urine, sweat, saliva, and gastric juice. By accelerating the exchange of sodium ions for potassium and hydrogen ions, aldosterone (the principal mineralocorticoid) produces a moderate potassium diuresis and increases the acidity of the urine. These renal effects of aldosterone help to regulate the concentration of potassium, hydrogen, and sodium ions in the blood—and this, in turn, affects the plasma volume.

In most species, a lack of mineralocorticoids is incompatible with life. The sodium loss that follows adrenalectomy leads, in the dog and in man, to circulatory insufficiency, hypotension, and eventually, fatal shock unless mineralocorticoids are supplied by replacement therapy.

Normally, the amounts of sex hormones (androgens and estrogens) secreted by the adrenal cortex are insignificant. Neoplasms and certain congenital enzyme deficiencies, however, may cause one or both adrenals to secrete large amounts of these hormones. Among the clinical effects are changes in the genitalia and alterations in a variety of secondary sex characteristics.

II. Surgical Procedure

For bilateral adrenalectomy, the midline abdominal incision (described in Chapter 6) is used. The flank incision commonly used for adrenalectomy in human patients allows adequate exposure of only one adrenal gland. Cranial extension of the midline incision may be necessary; if so, care should be taken to avoid incising the ventral border (crus) of the diaphragm.

When the abdominal cavity is entered, the intestines should be packed to one side with sterile, saline-moistened towels or sponges to allow adequate exposure of the perirenal area. Because of its proximity to the postcava, the right adrenal gland is usually more difficult to remove than the left; hence, most students prefer to begin with it.

The right adrenal gland can be located by palpation in the area around the cranial pole of the right kidney. It is usually found in the tissue beneath the postcava between the hilus of the kidney and the diaphragm. If the adrenal gland is located under the postcava, use careful blunt dissection to free the postcava from its peritoneal attachments. The postcava can then be retracted medially with closed Mixter forceps to provide adequate visualization of the right adrenal gland for its removal.

The phrenicoabdominal vein crosses over the middle of the right adrenal gland prior to entering the postcava. This vein can be dissected from the adrenal gland; however, the preferred method is to ligate it with 00 silk at its entry into the postcava and on the other side of the adrenal gland. The vein is then transected; the adrenal gland is dissected free from all surrounding fat and connective tissue, and removed.

The left adrenal gland is easier to remove surgically because it is not close to any major vessel except the phrenicoabdominal vein on its ventral surface. This vein is ligated and transected in the same way as described for the one on the right side. The adrenal gland is then bluntly dissected from its connective tissue attachments and removed.

When both of the adrenal glands have been removed the surgeon removes the sponges and checks the abdominal cavity for any other sponges or instruments that may have been left in the area. After inspecting the abdominal cavity for any abnormalities or signs of bleeding, the surgeon closes the incision in the manner previously described for a midline incision (Chapter 6).

III. Preoperative and Postoperative Care

A. Preoperative treatment

One day prior to surgery, the dog should receive 25 mg of cortisone acetate by intramuscular injection. This should be repeated on the day of surgery. In addition, the dog should receive 250–300 ml of 5% dextrose in saline i.v. during the surgical procedure, 100 mg of hydrocortisone sodium succinate i.v. after removal of the second adrenal gland, and 5 mg of desoxycorticosterone acetate intramuscularly after closing the incision.

This premedication will help to ensure capillary integrity and to prevent the shock which might result from the rapid and complete loss of adrenal function.

B. Postoperative care

In addition to the basic postsurgical care described in Chapter 6, the dog will require some initial adrenal cortical hormone treatment to recover from the surgical procedures. Give 25 mg of cortisone acetate (oral or intramuscular injection) or 10 mg of prednisone orally on day 1 postsurgically. No further hormone treatment should be given unless there are signs of an adrenal crisis.

C. Adrenal crisis

The proposed replacement therapy is based on average requirements and may be insufficient to meet the animal's needs for homeostasis. In such cases of acute adrenal insufficiency, the classic signs include anorexia, vomiting, bloody diarrhea, hypotension, restlessness, severe weakness, and lethargy. Ultimately, coma and circulatory collapse will ensue if treatment is not provided.

Replacement therapy in an adrenal crisis is directed at providing adequate adrenal cortical hormones and support of the cardiovascular system. The initial treatment should consist of:

1. 300 ml of 5% dextrose in saline i.v.
2. A total of 100 mg of cortisone acetate injected intramuscularly in two to four different sites.
3. 10 mg of desoxycorticosterone acetate injected intramuscularly

On the day following (12–24 hours) this treatment, the dog should be given:

1. 300 ml of 5% dextrose in saline i.v.
2. A total of 50 mg of cortisone acetate injected intramuscularly in one site
3. 10 mg of desoxycorticosterone pivalate injected intramuscularly

This treatment is then followed by 5 mg of prednisone orally each day for 6 days and every other day thereafter.

If the adrenal crisis is severe or the hypotension persists, the following treatment should be given:

1. 5% dextrose in saline intravenously as required (at least 300 ml)
2. 100 mg of hydrocortisone sodium succinate intravenously
3. 0.3 to 0.5 mg of phenylephrine hydrochloride subcutaneously every 1–2 hours until the blood pressure is maintained within normal limits.
4. 10 mg of desoxycorticosterone acetate injected intramuscularly

On the following day the dog should receive:

1. 300 ml of 5% dextrose in saline i.v.
2. 50 mg of cortisone acetate intramuscularly
3. 10 mg of desoxycorticosterone pivalate intramuscularly

This treatment is then followed by 5 mg of prednisone orally each day for 6 days and every other day thereafter.

D. Laboratory procedures

A minimum of 5 ml of blood should be collected on post-operative days 2, 5, 7, 9, and 14. An additional blood sample should be taken at the time of adrenal crisis, before replacement therapy is started. The serum from these samples is extracted and frozen at $-20°C$ until making determination of the glucose, sodium, potassium, and chloride content.

IV. Clinical Considerations

The lack of mineralocorticoids following removal of the adrenal glands causes sodium and chloride to be lost in the urine, with subsequent retention of potassium by the kidneys. Hence, the serum concentration of sodium and chloride decreases, while the concentration of potassium increases. A decrease in plasma ionic concentration following the loss of aldosterone secretion leads to a diminution of the plasma volume, with resultant hypotension, circulatory insufficiency, and eventually, fatal shock.

In experimental cases of adrenal insufficiency in the dog, the lack of glucocorticoids is not as life-threatening as the lack of mineralocorticoids. Since gluconeogenesis is responsible, in part, for maintaining the blood sugar at normal levels, the lack of gluco-corticoids can result in hypoglycemia, especially during periods of stress. This effect is much less pronounced in the dog than in man. In the dog, hypoglycemia occurs only in the terminal stages of adrenal insufficiency.

12

Parathyroidectomy and Thyroidectomy

C. MAX LANG AND WILLIAM J. WHITE

Parathyroidectomy (Gk. *para,* beyond; Gr. *thyreoeidēs,* shield-shaped; and Gk. *ektomē,* excision) refers to the surgical removal of the parathyroid glands.[1] Because of their close association with the thyroid glands, the thyroids are often removed during parathyroidectomy.

The experimental removal of these glands gives the student surgeon additional experience in endocrine surgery, as well as a demonstration of the role played by parathyroids in calcium and phosphorus metabolism.

I. Anatomy

A. Thyroid glands

The thyroid gland of the dog is composed of two separate lobes lying lateral to the first three tracheal rings (Figs. 42 and 43). In man, and in some dogs, the two lobes are connected by a glandular isthmus. In most dogs, however, the two lobes are connected by only a small sheet of fibrous tissue.

Location of the thyroid glands varies considerably among individuals and species. As a rule, the cranial pole of the right lobe lies opposite the first tracheal ring—one to two rings higher than

[1] Dorland's *Illustrated Medical Dictionary.* (1974). 25th ed. Philadelphia: W. B. Saunders Company.

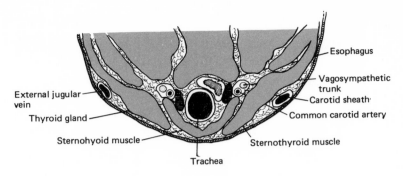

External jugular vein
Thyroid gland
Sternohyoid muscle
Trachea
Esophagus
Vagosympathetic trunk
Carotid sheath
Common carotid artery
Sternothyroid muscle

Fig. 42. Cross section of the ventral aspect of the canine neck at the level of the thyroid gland.

the cranial pole of the left lobe. Attachment of the lobes to the trachea is less intimate in the dog than in man. The lobes are well covered with fascia and are often as closely attached to the overlying musculature as to the trachea. The size and shape of the thyroid glands vary with the amount of iodine in the diet and with the level of estrogen secretion.

Like most endocrine glands, the thyroid is richly supplied with blood vessels and nerves; however, the size of these structures is so small that they are of little significance in this surgical procedure. In most dogs, the principal source of supply is the cranial thyroid artery, which gives off a number of small branches to each lobe. This vessel arises from the common carotid artery, just opposite the larynx, and runs caudally. Usually one large branch of this vessel continues caudally to the thoracic inlet, in close association with the recurrent laryngeal nerve. When a caudal thyroid artery is present, it may anastomose with this branch. Both caudal thyroid arteries, when present, arise from a common trunk of the brachiocephalic artery. These vessels, which may occasionally be the major source of supply to the glands, run cranially along either side of the trachea parallel to the recurrent laryngeal nerve.

Venous drainage of the thyroid glands is principally by the caudal thyroid vein, which arises from the caudal border of each lobe and empties into the internal jugular vein on that side. A cranial thyroid vein, which is a satellite of the cranial thyroid artery, also drains some of the venous blood from the cranial portions of the lobes.

The thyroid is innervated by fibers derived from the sympathetic components of the cranial cervical ganglion and from the cranial laryngeal nerve. In addition, vascular plexuses carry fibers from

114

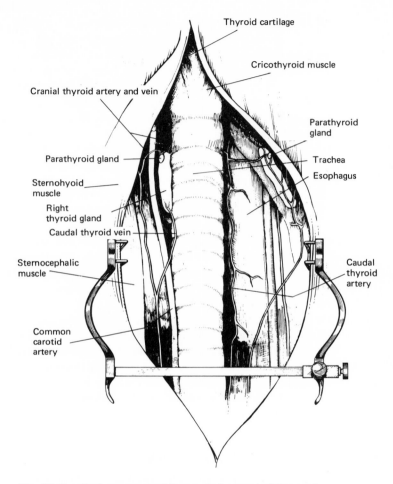

Fig. 43. Surgical exposure of the ventral aspect of the canine neck, showing thyroid and parathyroid glands with surrounding structures.

the caudal cervical ganglia to the thyroid gland. Direct innervation of the thyroid gland is of little importance, since pituitary hormones and changes in blood flow are the principal mechanisms for controlling thyroid secretion.

B. Parathyroid glands

The parathyroid glands are small, oval bodies directly associated with each thyroid gland. They vary in location and number between individuals and species. Most dogs have four parathyroid glands—two attached to each thyroid. The glands are often named according to their location with respect to the thyroid. Those located on the lateral surface of the thyroid (commonly in connective tissue at the cranial pole of each lobe) are termed *external;* those embedded on the medial surface of the caudal pole are termed *internal.* Since the external glands are derived from the third pharyngeal pouch and the internal glands from the fourth, the two sets of glands may also be referred to as *parathyroids III and IV.*

As a rule, the external parathyroid glands are separated from the capsule of the thyroid by a connective tissue septum and have a separate blood supply—a branch from the cranial thyroid artery. Thus, it is possible to remove the thyroid gland without removing the external parathyroids. The internal parathyroid glands, on the other hand, lie underneath the capsule of the thyroid gland and are often firmly embedded in the parenchyma. They are nourished by branches arising from the thyroid parenchyma. It is, therefore, impossible to remove the thyroid without removing the internal parathyroid gland.

Both internal and external parathyroids share the venous and lymphatic drainage of the thyroid gland.

In some species, total parathyroidectomy is occasionally complicated by the presence of accessory parathyroid tissue. These accessory glands may be found within the thyroid, associated with the thymus gland, or in the region of the larynx, carotid sheath, or anterior mediastinum.

II. Physiology of the Parathyroid Glands

The parathyroid glands secrete *parathormone*—a substance which increases the urinary excretion of phosphate, raises plasma calcium levels by mobilizing calcium stored in bone, and increases the absorption of calcium from the intestine. The output of parathormone varies inversely with the concentration of calcium in the plasma.

Most of the body's calcium exists in pools within the bones: a readily exchangeable pool, which is in equilibrium with the plasma; and a slowly exchangeable pool, which releases stored calcium very gradually. In the absence of parathormone, the former pool can maintain the plasma calcium concentration at 4–6 mg/100 ml; but such concentrations are usually incompatible with life. Normal plasma calcium concentrations (9–11 mg/100 ml) can be maintained only if parathormone is present in normal quantities.

Parathormone is a single-chain polypeptide with a molecular weight of approximately 8000 and a relatively short biologic half-life. Although some of the intact hormone is excreted in the urine, little is known about the metabolism of the compound, or about the mechanism of action whereby it increases the concentration of calcium in the serum. It has been reported that parathormone may stimulate DNA-dependent RNA synthesis, and it has been shown that parathormone causes an increase in the plasma concentration of citrates. One theory is that a high concentration of citrates in the extracellular fluid of bone binds calcium and, thus, lowers the local concentration of calcium ions so that more bone calcium goes into solution. Citric acid also increases the solubility of calcium by decreasing the pH of the extracellular fluid.

The action of parathormone is not limited to the release of calcium from the bone. By increasing the secretion of phosphate ions through the renal tubules, it causes a decrease in plasma phosphate. Among the other reported effects of parathormone are its abilities to increase the intestinal absorption of calcium and to increase the mitochondrial uptake of certain inorganic ions, for example, magnesium, phosphate, and potassium.

III. Surgical Procedure

Both the thyroid and the parathyroid glands are removed through a midline incision on the ventral surface of the neck (Fig. 44). The purpose of removing the thyroid gland is to ensure complete removal of the internal parathyroids. Skillful blunt dissection and careful hemostasis will be required if all glandular structures are to be seen.

The dog is placed in the dorsal recumbent position with the neck extended (Fig. 44). Adhesive tape may be used to keep the head in place on the table. Folded towels beneath the neck may be needed to elevate and support it. The neck is then clipped from the thoracic inlet to a point 5 cm anterior to the ramus of the mandible (Fig. 44). After preparation of the skin, the area is draped. To ensure that the incision is correctly placed, the larynx, trachea, and thoracic inlet should be palpated through the drape.

Beginning 1½ to 2 cm anterior to the caudal border of the larynx on the ventral midline, a skin incision is made and extended

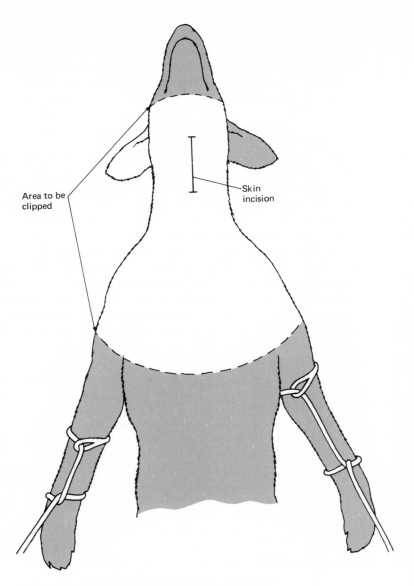

Fig. 44. Site of the incision for parathyroidectomy.

caudally for 10 cm using a #20 scalpel in a #4 handle. The incision is continued through the fascial layers until the underlying sternohyoid muscle is exposed, running in a cranial-caudal direction. Blunt dissection is used to separate these muscle fibers, thus, exposing the underlying trachea. With the fibers of the sternohyoid retracted to either side, the first four tracheal rings are located by palpation. At this level, blunt dissection is continued laterally on either side of the trachea, underneath the sternohyoid muscle. The fibers of this muscle run in a cranial-caudal direction at a 45° angle to the median plane.

The almond-shaped thyroid gland, covered with connective tissue, will be found lying dorsal and somewhat lateral to the trachea. They are bordered laterally by the carotid sheath; the left is bordered medially by the esophagus, the right by the trachea. In consistency, it resembles a lymph node. While each thyroid gland is being bluntly dissected away from the connective tissue, an attempt should be made to locate the external parathyroid glands. Otherwise, they may be inadvertently separated from the capsule of the thyroid and, thus, left in the body.

If it is necessary to ligate any of the thyroid blood vessels, the ligatures should be placed far enough away from the parenchyma of the gland to ensure that no parathyroid tissue is included in the ligature. Blunt dissection and ligation should be continued until each lobe of the thyroid can be removed. After removal, both lobes should be inspected for the presence of external and internal parathyroid glands.

In order to decrease dead space under the muscles when the incision is closed, a few simple interrupted 00 chromic surgical gut sutures should be used to pull the muscle fibers down onto the deeper fascial planes. Care should be taken not to incorporate the trachea, carotid sheath, or esophagus in any of these sutures. The separated fibers of the sternohyoid muscle may be apposed by a few simple interrupted sutures of 00 chromic surgical gut. A continuous line of subcutaneous sutures of 00 chromic surgical gut is used to appose the skin edges and decrease dead space. Simple interrupted sutures of nonabsorbable suture material should be used to close the skin.

IV. Postsurgical Care

The basic postoperative care is the same as that described in Chapter 6.

The dog should be examined at least twice daily, at which time its respiratory rate, heart rate, muscle tone, reflexes, and degree of activity should be recorded. Preoperatively and on postoperative days 2, 6, and 10, 5 ml of blood should be collected in a clot tube for calcium and phosphorus determinations.

When signs of tetany develop—whether before or after all the postoperative samples have been taken—an additional sample should be collected before any medication or dietary change is initiated. Then approximately 0.5 gm of calcium chloride or calcium gluconate solution is slowly given intravenously until the signs of tetany subside. Two hours after the signs of tetany abate, another blood sample is withdrawn for calcium and phosphorus determinations.

V. Clinical Considerations

Although loss of thyroid function can have serious consequences (myxedema), the signs of parathyroid deficiency appear more rapidly and are more acute. Parathormone is essential to life. Inadequate levels of the hormone lead to hypocalcemia and the clinical syndrome known as *hypocalcemic tetany.* This condition develops rapidly following total parathyroidectomy. The signs— listlessness, anorexia, vomiting, subnormal temperature, tachycardia, muscular excitability, muscular fasiculations, local or general muscle spasms, laryngospasm, and exaggerated (hyperactive) reflexes—usually appear 2 to 5 days after the operation. Another sign that may occur is a marked increase in the respiratory rate, which becomes identical with the heart rate. This phenomenon is due to stimulation of the phrenic nerve by electrical impulses radiating from the heart during systole.

Calcium is necessary for normal muscle contraction, nerve function, and blood coagulation. When extracellular fluid levels of calcium are decreased, the transmission of impulses at the myoneural junction is inhibited. The hypocalcemic tetany seen clinically is a central nervous system effect produced by the lack of free ionized calcium in the extracellular tissue fluids. This is contrary to popular opinion that the muscular symptoms are produced by local stimulation of muscles resulting from decreased calcium levels in the peripheral blood.

Although blood coagulation is also dependent upon calcium (which acts as a cofactor in several of the enzymatic steps necessary to convert fibrinogen to fibrin), bleeding seldom occurs until the serum calcium level drops below 4 mg/100 ml.

13

Laminectomy

HOWARD C. HUGHES, JR., AND C. MAX LANG

Laminectomy (L. *lamina,* layer; and Gk. *ektomē,* excision) is defined as "surgical removal of one or more laminas of the vertebrae, often including the spinous processes of the vertebrae."[1] Clinically this technique is used to relieve pressure on the spinal cord caused by a variety of processes, including calcification or rupture of intervertebral disks, spinal dislocation or fracture, and extradural hemorrhage.

There are two types of laminectomies: dorsal laminectomy and hemilaminectomy. The former involves removal of the entire dorsal lamina of the vertebra; in the latter, half of the dorsal arch is removed.

I. Anatomy of the Vertebrae

For an appreciation of the differences between the two procedures, a knowledge of vertebral anatomy is essential. Although each type of vertebra is somewhat different, a lumbar vertebra is shown in Fig. 45 for demonstration purposes. A typical vertebra consists of a body and an arch, the latter being formed by two pedicles and two laminas. The arch supports nine processes—four articular, two transverse, two accessory, and one spinous. The

---

[1] *Dorland's Illustrated Medical Dictionary.* (1974). 25th ed. Philadelphia: W. B. Saunders Co.

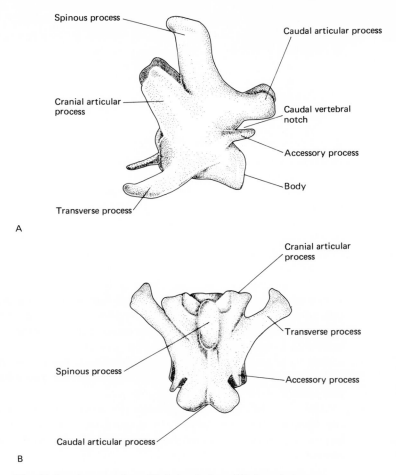

Fig. 45. Lumbar vertebra. (A) Lateral view; (B) dorsal view.

spinous process is a single midline projection arising from the dorsal aspect of the vertebra and sloping forward. The *articular processes* lie lateral to the midline, the caudal articular processes of one vertebra extending between the cranial articular processes of the vertebra below. The *transverse processes* arise from the lateral aspects of the vertebral body and extend ventrocranially. All of the processes are sites for the attachment of ligaments and muscles needed to keep the spinal column in proper alignment.

The intervertebral disks are located between the bodies of apposing vertebrae. These structures form the articulations between vertebrae and serve as cushioning mechanisms against forces traveling along the axis of the spinal column.

II. Surgical Procedure

The instructor should assign a different lumbar vertebra to each group of students, so that the students can see the effects of cord or nerve-root lesions at different levels.

The anesthetized dog is placed in ventral recumbency. A sand bag may be placed under the neck to elevate the surgical site. The skin incision is made in the dorsal midline, using a #20 blade in a #4 handle. The incision should be 12–15 cm long, with the center over the vertebra assigned for laminectomy. With a #10 blade in a #3 handle, the dorsal fascia is incised to expose the sacrospinalis muscles. The muscle is bluntly dissected away from the spinous and articular processes, so that the dorsal body of the vertebra and the intervertebral space can be seen. If a dorsal laminectomy is being performed, the muscle on each side of the spinous process is removed; if the operation is a hemilaminectomy, the muscle is removed only on one side.

For a *hemilaminectomy,* a pair of rongeur forceps is used to remove the articular process over the intervertebral space. To enter the spinal canal, a laminectomy trephine is gently but firmly rotated in a clockwise direction until the lamina gives way under the pressure. The trephine with its plug of bone is then gently removed, and the rongeur forceps are used to enlarge the hole by carefully removing small pieces of bone from the inside edge.

For a *dorsal laminectomy,* the spinous process is removed along with the articular process, so that the entire dorsal surface of the cord is exposed. The dorsal lamina is then carefully removed from the cord with a laminectomy trephine or a high-speed drill. Sufficient vertebrae should be removed so that the nerve root is easily visualized. Care must always be taken in extending the laminectomy, since the cord is easily damaged. Injury or damage to the cord is evident since the animal's body jumps or twitches caudal to the laminectomy site when an instrument touches the cord. This "jump" is a result of the massive discharge of the dorsal root neurons.

Carefully, pick up the nerve root with a nerve hook just before it exits through the vertebral body. Examine it prior to transection for any vessels which might be entering the cord along with the root. The distribution of these vessels is highly variable and no set pattern of anatomic distribution exists. Cut the nerve roots with Metzenbaum scissors. If a vessel is present, double ligate it with the root prior to transection.

Closure of the wound is the same for both types of laminectomies. The sacrospinalis muscles are sutured with 00 chromic surgical gut so as to eliminate all dead space, and the fascia is closed in a similar manner. Simple interrupted nonabsorbable sutures may be used to close the skin incision.

III. Postsurgical Care

Depending upon the degree and extent of the spinal injury, it may be necessary to administer physical therapy in addition to the basic care described in Chapter 6. One of the best forms of physical therapy is hydrotherapy. The dog is placed in a large tub of water so that its legs do not touch the bottom. Supported by the water, the animal is able to exercise the affected limbs without the stress of weight-bearing.

In some cases bandages or prosthetic devices may be necessary to prevent decubitus sores or injury resulting from denervation of one or more limbs. In cases where the sympathetic nerve system has been damaged, an indwelling catheter may be necessary to relieve urinary stasis, and enemas may be required to prevent fecal impaction.

IV. Clinical Considerations

A. Comparison of both types of laminectomies

Both types of laminectomies are used clinically to provide decompression following injuries causing pressure on the spinal cord. The major disadvantages of the dorsal laminectomy are (1) inability to visualize the ventral surface of the cord, especially if removal of the disk is required; and (2) the greater risk of surgical and postoperative trauma created by exposure of such a large area of the cord.

The hemilaminectomy allows for both decompression and visualization of the ventral surface of the cord. Its major disadvantage is the possibility of severe hemorrhage if the venous sinus is entered.

B. Neurologic examination

Through the use of relatively simple methods of testing, the effects of nerve root sectioning or spinal cord injury can be evaluated. The neurologic examination is centered on (1) motor pathways, (2) sensory pathways, and (3) reflex arches. It should be remembered that in conducting a neurologic examination, patient cooperation is extremely important. Calm, firm, and quiet mannerism on the examiner's part are imperative.

Motor abnormalities are best detected by observing the animal's movements. If the animal is able to walk, the examiner should observe his gait. These voluntary motor movements are classified as normal, weak (paretic), or absent (paralysis). An attempt should be made to characterize the movement deficit as a function of muscle groups.

Knuckling over is a test of conscious proprioception. If necessary, support the animal under its abdomen and knuckle over the foot, that is, turn the paw over so that the dorsal surface is on the floor. A normal dog will immediately replace its foot in a normal position. A delay of 5 seconds is classified as a weak response. Delays for longer periods usually indicate a complete loss of proprioception.

Sensory loss is determined with the pinprick test. Starting at the tail end and working forward, the skin is carefully and systematically pricked with a large safety pin. (Small pins or needles should not be used since they will puncture the skin). If the prick is felt, the animal will usually turn its head in recognition. The skin may also twitch due to movement of subcutaneous muscle, however, this is a reflex and does not indicate an intact sensory system.

Deep pain can be demonstrated by squeezing the feet, tendons, or testis. If superficial sensory preception is intact, there is no point in doing the deep pain examination. With deep pain the animal should also show an indication of recognition of the deep pain by crying out or attempts to escape. Withdrawal of the leg alone is a simple spinal reflex and does not indicate a conscious response.

Further examination of the spinal reflexes will aid in the localization of the lesion. The basic reflexes to be examined are the knee jerk, flexor withdrawal, extensor thrust, and the anal. As shown in Table II each of these reflexes requires that certain nerves be present and functioning normally.

The knee jerk requires that the femoral nerve, spinal nerves L4 through L6, and the spinal cord itself from L3 to L5 be intact and functioning properly. The knee jerk is tested by sharply strik-

Table II   Lumbar nerves comprising the lumbosacral plexus and their areas of innervation

Lumbar nerve root	Lumbar nerve	Innervation
1	Cranial iliohypogastric	Muscles and skin of
2	Caudal iliohypogastric	caudolateral abdo-
3	Ilioinguinal	men wall; skin of lateral thigh in knee region.
3, 4	External spermatic	Sensory to prepuce, scrotum, and skin on dorsal medial surface of thigh.
4	Lateral cutaneous	Sensory to cranial lateral surface of thigh.
4, 5, 6	Femoral	Sensory to medial surface of thigh, knee, leg, and foot; motor to quadriceps group, iliopsoas and sartorius muscles.
5, 6 ˙	Obturator	Motor to external obturator, pectineus, abductor and gracilis muscles.
6, 7, S_1	Sciatic	Sensory to caudal and lateral surface of thigh, craniolateral and caudal surfaces of lower leg; motor to flexor muscles of knee, extensor muscles of tarsus, extensors and flexors of digits.

ing the patellar tendon of the flexed knee with a rubber neurologic hammer. A positive response is the immediate extension of the knee due to contraction of the quadraceps muscle group.

The withdrawal reflex for the hind leg tests the function of the sciatic nerve, nerve roots L6, L7, and S1, and the spinal cord segments in the last three lumbar vertebrae. This reflex is tested by firmly squeezing the toes or foot pad. A positive response is the flexion of the leg. A positive withdrawal reflex may be present with spinal cord injury above L5. In this case, it may also elicit a crossed extensor response; as the one foot is squeezed and withdrawn the opposite leg extends.

The extensor thrust reflex is tested for by simply putting upward pressure on the bottom of the foot. Resistance to flexion of the leg should be felt and the animal will straighten its leg. This reflex is required for the animal to stand, however, with a high cord lesion it is possible to have spasticity. This may produce extensor rigidity, resulting in the legs becoming stiff and straight. At times, it is possible, with extensor rigidity, to stand the animal in an upright position. Proprioception, however, is absent and the animal will fall over when movement is attempted.

Anal reflexes and bladder control are mediated by the sacral nerves. Pinpricking around the anus should elicit sphincter constriction indicating the functional integrity of the cord and nerve roots supplying this area.

These reflexes should be tested preoperatively as well as daily following the surgery. The cutting of only one nerve root will not affect an entire nerve because each nerve arises from three or more roots. Minor deficits, however, in both sensory and reflex functions on the side of the severance will be visible immediately postoperatively. These neurologic deficits, provided there is no spinal cord damage, are usually transitory with improvement being visible on a daily basis. This improvement will continue for 3 to 7 days after which the animal will appear functionally normal. Only a small area of sensory deficit may remain.

If spinal cord damage is suspected, one should continue with a more complete neurologic examination involving more sensory and proprioceptive responses. These are described in Chapter 14 and are used to determine the integrity of the nervous system between the brain and spinal cord.

14

Ablation of the Motor Cortex

HOWARD C. HUGHES, JR., AND C. MAX LANG

Various types of neuropathology can be simulated experimentally by creating surgical lesions in certain areas of the brain. While the motor and sensory deficits that result are related to the specific area of the brain that has been damaged, the ablation of portions of the motor cortex in dogs will not always produce obvious motor deficiencies. In the dog and other vertebrates, other regions of the brain also contribute to motor performance and may compensate for the cortical damage.

I. Anatomy of the Brain

Through a series of divisions, the brain develops from the rostral (intracranial) portion of the neural tube into its final form, with three principal divisions: the cerebrum, the brain stem, and the cerebellum. The cerebrum is subdivided into two hemispheres, each of which is considered to have four topographical areas, called lobes: frontal, parietal, occipital, and temporal. The cerebral cortex consists of an outer layer of gray matter and an inner, or medullary, area of white matter. The surface of the brain is not smooth but is extensively folded in a fairly consistent pattern; therefore, surface features such as *sulci* (grooves, or depressions) and *gyri* (elevations, or convolutions) can be used as landmarks to demarcate specific areas of the cortex.

The area of interest in this procedure is found on either side of a

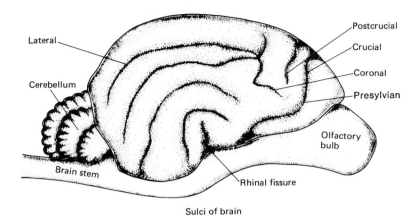

Sulci of brain

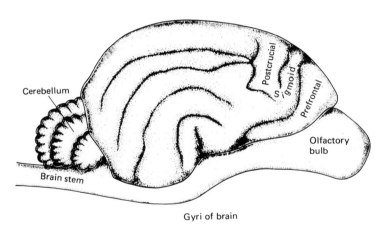

Gyri of brain

Fig. 46. Lateral view of the canine brain.

conspicuous sulcus, the *crucial sulcus,* located on the dorsal aspect of
the cerebrum (Fig. 46). The crucial sulcus is completely sur-
rounded by the *sigmoid gyrus* (Fig. 46), which in turn is bordered
by *presylvian sulcus* cranially, the *coronal sulcus* ventrally, and the
postcrucial sulcus caudally.

Electrical stimulation of selected cortical areas has determined
that the motor area lies in the vicinity of the sigmoid and postcrucial gyri. This motor area contains a large number of giant
pyramidal, or Betz, cells which form the axons of the corticospinal
tract.

II. Surgical Procedure

The dog should be placed in the sternal recumbent position with its head extended and elevated by a sandbag. The skin over the entire calvarium is clipped, scrubbed, and swabbed with an antiseptic solution. (Care should be taken to prevent the fluids from entering the eyes.) After the area is draped, a scalpel with a #20 blade in a #4 handle is used to make a midline incision from the level of the supraorbital process to the occipital protuberance. The skin over one temporal muscle is bluntly dissected away from the muscle and retracted. The attachments of the temporal muscle lie about 1–3 mm from the midline. After these have been palpated, a scalpel with a #10 blade in a #3 handle is used to cut the overlying temporal fascia about 3 mm from its attachment to the calvarium. The muscle is then bluntly dissected from the bone and reflected ventrally.

The site where the calvarium is to be entered lies at the junction of two imaginary lines—one drawn 1 cm lateral to the midline, and the other from the lateral canthus of the eye to the auditory canal (Fig. 47). The bone is carefully removed from this area with a trephine or a drill, and the hole is then enlarged with a pair of rongeur forceps. This procedure should expose the crucial sulcus. The surgeon should be careful to remove all bone fragments from the incision. Bone wax may be used to control bleeding from the bone.

A scalpel with a #11 blade in a #3 handle is used to make an incision in the dura, which is reflected away from the sulcus. Care must be taken to avoid incising the dorsal sagittal sinus, which lies in the falx cerebri; cutting into this venous sinus will result in uncontrollable hemorrhage.

With a suction apparatus, the gray matter is removed from the sigmoid gyrus and the rostral half of the postcrucial gyrus. The surgeon should avoid entering the lateral ventricle. Minor cerebral hemorrhage can be controlled with gelatin sponges.

After the ablation is complete, the dura is replaced but not necessarily sutured. The temporal muscle is also replaced, and the fascia is sutured with 00 chromic surgical gut to the 3 mm strip left on the calvarium. The bone cannot be replaced, but the bone defect will repair itself.

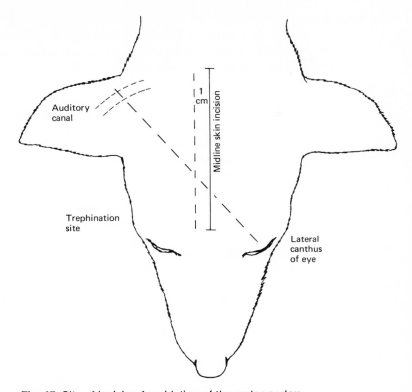

Fig. 47. Site of incision for ablation of the motor cortex.

III. Neurologic Examination

In order to evaluate the extent of the neurologic deficit created, a complete neurologic examination must be done before and after surgery. Like any procedure requiring cooperation on the patient's part, a neurologic examination must be performed in a firm, calm manner. Loud noises, sudden movements, and impatience will excite the animal and make evaluation of the neurologic reflexes difficult if not impossible.

A. Observation of gait

The first and most important aspect of any examination involving motor function is evaluation of the subject's gait. The examiner should observe the dog from the front and the side while he is running and walking. Defects in gait will be produced by motor deficiencies ranging from loss of function in a single muscle to paresis of whole muscle groups and even limbs.

B. Testing of reflexes

Some motor deficiencies can be detected only by examination of certain neurologic reflexes. A lesion in the motor cortex has no effect on the *spinal reflexes:* the patellar reflex, flexor-withdraw reflex, anal reflex, and extensor thrust reflex. The *proprioceptive* (postural and attitudinal) *reflexes,* however, require an intact central nervous system. In order to test these reflexes, it may be necessary to cover the dog's eyes; otherwise, the animal's response to visual stimuli may create a false impression that the proprioceptive reflexes are intact.

The *placing reaction* is a postural reflex involving movement of the front limbs to support the animal's weight. The technique for assessing this reflex is as follows: With the animal on the table, the left hand is placed under his chin to keep the head raised, and the right hand is placed under his chest so that the forelegs are raised off the ground and swing freely. When the dorsa of the forelegs are allowed to touch the edge of the table, a normal dog will immediately raise his feet and place them firmly on the table.

The *righting reflex* is a postural reflex used to assess the animal's motor coordination. This reflex may be elicited by holding the dog upside down over a padded surface and dropping him. (He should be dropped from a point high enough to allow him ample space to turn over and land on his feet before striking the surface.) When the righting reflex is intact the animal will land on his feet in an upright position. A safer way to test this is holding the animal down on his side or back or watching him right himself when released. Normal animals will quickly scramble to their feet; but animals with motor-cortex lesions will be much slower. The righting reflex may also be depressed in the presence of vestibular lesions.

The *extensor postural thrust* is another reflex which is commonly used to evaluate lesions of the cerebellum, vestibular apparatus, and spinal cord. This reflex depends on the integrity of the motor pathways and the central nervous system. To elicit this reflex, the animal's front legs are raised off the floor and moved forward. When they are lowered to the floor, the dog's hind limbs should move forward to support his weight.

The *hopping reflex* is used to evaluate the animal's ability to correct the position of his front limbs. To elicit this reflex, both hind legs and one front leg are held off the floor. The other front leg is left in contact with a firm surface, and is bearing part of the animal's weight. If the hopping reflex is intact, the dog should be able to keep its leg under it in a supporting position as he is moved forward, backward, or sideways.

The use of these tests and observations will help the student to assess the extent and severity of the lesion in the motor cortex. It is important to remember that decussation of the nerves causes cerebral defects to be manifested on the contralateral side of the body.

All of these reflexes should be tested before surgery and on the second, fourth, and sixth postoperative days. Since the dog has a relatively diffuse motor cortical area, neurologic deficits which are pronounced a few days after surgery may diminish as lower centers begin to take over the function of the motor cortex.

Laboratory Techniques

The following chapters describe certain basic laboratory procedures often used to evaluate the patient's postoperative course
and the effects of surgery. When interpreting the results of these
procedures, however, the student surgeon must bear in mind that
all animals (and man) have a certain degree of biologic variability.
Normal values for clinical laboratory tests vary greatly with the
species, and also with the method of analysis and even the
laboratory in which they are performed.

15

Clinical Laboratory Methods in Physiologic Surgery

WILLIAM J. WHITE AND C. MAX LANG

Clinical laboratory determinations are often essential to the clinician, both in confirming a diagnosis and in developing a prognosis. For the student performing surgical procedures outlined in this text, laboratory determinations are often necessary to follow the animal's postoperative course and in determining whether the surgical goal of producing a given syndrome has been achieved.

The laboratory methods needed for this course in physiologic surgery are described in the following section. Where possible, guidelines for interpreting the results of these tests are included. Normal values for the dog are presented in Tables III and IV.

I. Sample Collection

The proper collection, preservation, and preparation of whole blood or its components are important preliminaries to any clinical laboratory determination. The accuracy as well as the validity of these determinations depends in large measure on properly prepared specimens that are suitable for the analytic procedure. Before collecting any sample, the student surgeon should consult Table V.

A. Types of samples

Serum is the fluid portion of blood devoid of those factors used in the formation of a clot. Plasma is serum that still contains all the elements necessary for clot formation. Whole blood contains

Table III   Normative data for the dog: Hematology

	Range	*(Average)*
Total RBC (per mm³)	5.5– 8.5 × 10⁶	6.8 × 10⁶
Total WBC (per mm³)	6.0–17.0 × 10³	11.5 × 10³

Leukocyte counts	*Relative (%)*		*Absolute (per mm³)*	
	Range	*Average*	*Range*	*Average*
Neutrophils (PMN's)	60–77	70	3,000–11,500	7000
Bands (immature PMN's)	0– 3	0.8	0– 300	70
Lymphocytes	12–30	20	1,000– 4,000	2800
Monocytes	3–10	5.2	150– 1,350	750
Eosinophils	2–10	4.0	100– 1,250	550
Basophils	Rare	0.0	Rare	0.0
Hematocrit (PCV) (%)	37–55	45		
Hemoglobin (Hb) (gm/100 ml)	12–18	15		

Table IV   Normative data for the dog: Clinical chemistry

	Normal Values
Urea nitrogen (BUN)	10 – 20 mg/100 ml
Calcium	8.1– 12.2 mg/100 ml
Chloride	108 –119 mEq/L
Creatine phosphokinase (CPK)	12 –144 I.U.
Creatinine	1.0– 1.7 mg/100 ml
Glucose	55 – 90 mg/100 ml
Lactic dehydrogenase (LDH)	
Total	10 –126 I.U.
Isoenzymes (%)	
LDH₁	23.8 ± 11.1
LDH₂	11.1 ± 3.6
LDH₃	21.6 ± 4.9
LDH₄	12.6 ± 4.9
LDH₅	30.7 ± 13.7
α-Hydroxybutyrate dehydrogenase	14 – 62 I.U.
Phosphorus	2.2 – 4.0 mg/100 ml
Potassium	3.7 – 5.8 mEq/L
Sodium	140 –154 mEq/L
Blood pH	7.31– 7.42
p_{CO_2}	40 ± 5 torr
p_{O_2}	85 ± 5 torr

Table V   Stability of samples for clinical chemistry determinations

Laboratory determination[1]	Room Temperature (25° C)	4° C	−20° C
BUN	24 hours	Several days	6 months
Calcium	24 hours	Several days	7 days
Chloride	7 days	7 days	Indefinite
CPK	24 hours	5 days	7 days
Creatinine	5 days	24 hours	Indefinite
Glucose	1–24 hours	24 hours	24 hours
LDH (total, isoenzymes, and αHBD)	5 days	0	0
Phosphorus	Slight increase occurs on standing for 2 hours	7 days	Indefinite
Sodium and potassium	14 days	14 days	Indefinite
Blood-gas analysis[2]	5 minutes	1 hour	0

[1] All determinations except pH and blood gases require serum.

[2] This determination requires heparinized whole blood.

cellular elements as well as plasma. Clinical chemistry values are expressed in terms of amount per unit volume of blood or serum. Since clotting factors and cellular elements interfere with any chemical reactions, and since chemical constituents of blood are usually dissolved in the fluid portion, serum is the material utilized by most chemical tests. The concentration of chemical constituents in the serum is assumed to be equal to their concentration in whole blood, and the words blood, plasma, and serum are often used interchangeably in giving clinical chemistry values. Actually, the true blood concentration is somewhat lower than the serum concentration, since the serum determinations do not take into consideration the volume displaced by the cellular components and clotting factors in blood.

B. Drawing blood

The procedure of collecting and preparing samples should be carried out as quickly as possible, since blood from most species clots rapidly; and clotted blood is unsuitable for determinations which require whole blood. Hemolysis also makes the blood unsuitable for many tests, especially certain enzyme and electrolyte determinations. Hemolysis may be caused by: (1) contamination of the needle, syringe, or specimen tubes with water or with a sterilizing agent (for example, alcohol); (2) excessive temperatures (freezing or heating the specimen); (3) expulsion of blood from a syringe into the specimen tubes too rapidly; (4) failure to remove the needle before the blood is expelled; (5) undue delay before separating cells from the serum.

C. Preserving whole blood

When whole blood is used for an analysis, anticoagulants are needed to prevent clotting. Whole blood is required for complete blood counts (total red and while cell counts, differential, hematocrit, and hemoglobin) and for the determination of blood pH, p_{CO_2}, or p_{O_2}. Because it does not alter pH, p_{CO_2}, or p_{O_2}, the sodium or lithium salt of heparin is the preferred anticoagulant for samples to be used for determining blood gases. For hematologic determinations, the preferred anticoagulant is generally the disodium or dipotassium salt of ethylenediaminetetraacetic acid (EDTA). This anticoagulant should never be used with blood drawn for electrolyte determinations, since it binds many of the electrolytes normally present in the blood. EDTA will preserve blood for morphologic studies for a period of up to 8 hours.

Most of the clinical chemistry determinations called for in the preceding surgical exercises require serum rather than whole blood. Serum is prepared by placing whole blood in a dry, clean test tube without anticoagulant and allowing it to clot. After 15 to 30 minutes, the clot is loosened from the walls of the tube with an applicator stick and the tube is centrifuged at 2500 rpm for 10 minutes. The supernatant (serum) is then transferred immediately to a clean, dry tube by means of a transfer pipet. If it should be accidentally contaminated with red blood cells, the serum must be recentrifuged with red blood cells, and transferred to another clean, dry tube. The serum tube should be corked and labeled with the animal's number and the date of collection.

II. Hematology

A. Erythrocytes (red blood cells)

The erythrocyte component of the blood is evaluated by the means of the total red cell count, differential smear, hemoglobin, and hematocrit determinations. Although very little blood is required for any one of these determinations, it is a good idea to collect 3 to 5 ml of unclotted whole blood in EDTA to ensure sufficient blood for repeated determinations.

1. *Total red blood cell count (RBC)*

Because of its relative inaccuracy, the RBC is seldom performed. Essentially the same information can be obtained from calculations utilizing the hemoglobin and packed cell volume. The total red cell count is determined with a hemocytometer similar to the one used for the total white cell count. Because the number of cells counted per determination is so small in comparison to the number of red blood cells present in each aliquot of blood, errors in excess of 20% are common, even with experienced technicians.

2. *Differential count*

The differential smear is utilized to observe the size, shape, and morphologic characteristics of the erythrocytes. The presence of small erythrocytes (microcytosis), large erythrocytes (macrocytosis), distorted erythrocytes (leptocytosis), or nucleated erythrocytes (immature cells) can all be determined from the differential smear—as can variations in the size (anisocytosis) and shape (poikilocytosis) of the cells.

The differential smear is prepared by streaking a thin film of blood onto a clean glass microscope slide, air-drying it, and staining it with one of the Romanovsky stains (for example, Wright's stain). The staining characteristics of all blood elements should be noted during microscopic examination of the smear. Differences in the intensity of staining may cause the red cells to appear lighter or darker than normal (hypochromasia or hyperchromasia, respectively). The former condition may be due to a decrease in the concentration of hemoglobin or in the thickness of the red cells. Hyperchromasia is usually due to an increase in the thickness of the cells.

3. *Hemoglobin (Hb)*

Hemoglobin, the oxygen-carrying pigment of the blood, is found almost exclusively in the red blood cells. When used in conjunction with other parameters such as the differential smear and the hematocrit, determination of the hemoglobin concentration in whole blood can be quite useful in the diagnosis and classification of anemia and other blood disorders.

The methods commonly used for measuring the hemoglobin concentration of the blood are based on spectral characteristics of hemoglobin or its derivatives. Of these methods, the cyanmethemoglobin method is probably the one most widely used. This method involves converting the hemoglobin in a sample of blood to cyanmethemoglobin, which has an absorption peak at 540 nm. The concentration of hemoglobin in the sample is determined by reading aliquots of the sample in a spectrophotometer at 540 nm and comparing its absorbance to the absorbance of standard solutions of hemoglobin treated in a similar fashion.

4. *Hematocrit (packed cell volume, PCV)*

Determination of the hematocrit (volume percent of erythrocytes per unit of whole blood) requires that a sample of blood be centrifuged at high speed, so that the red blood cells are packed into the bottom of the container. Separating the layer of red blood cells from the plasma (or serum) portion of the blood is a thin layer of white cells. If a container of uniform shape and diameter is used, the volume of the red blood cells (PCV) can be easily measured and expressed as a percentage of the entire sample volume. The ease with which this test may be done makes it a very popular and sometimes overused clinical tool.

The hematocrit is dependent not only upon the number of red cells but also upon their size and the animal's state of hydration. It is conceivable that small numbers of large cells would occupy the same volume as large numbers of small cells. Furthermore, dehydration can cause a decrease in the volume of plasma and a misleading increase in the hematocrit.

B. Leukocytes

The leukocyte component of the blood is evaluated by means of the total white cell count and the differential smear. Interpretation of changes in the leukocyte component requires a knowledge of the normal distribution of leukocytes in the peripheral blood and the response of different cell types to disease. Accurate interpretation of leukocyte reactions, as expressed by changes in the distribution of different forms within the blood, can yield valuable information concerning the severity, duration, and prognosis of disease.

1. *Total white blood cell count (WBC)*

The WBC is extremely useful in indicating the presence of a variety of conditions, including infectious and/or inflammatory processes, toxemia, and physiologic stress. The total white cell count is often used in conjunction with the relative leukocyte distribution (obtained from the differential smear) to determine the absolute numbers of specific types of white cells. This information is helpful in determining whether abnormal populations of one or more leukocyte types are present when the total numbers of white cells are increased (leukocytosis). Increased numbers of cells are indicated by the suffixes *-ia* and *-osis*. The suffix *-penia* indicates an abnormally small number of cells.

The total number of white cells per cubic millimeter of blood is determined in the following manner. An aliquot of whole blood is diluted with a chemical solution which lyses red blood cells but leaves the leukocytes intact. After being thoroughly mixed, this mixture is used to fill a special ruled chamber on a microscope slide calibrated to hold a precise volume of solution. This special microscope slide, called a hemocytometer, has a number of ruled squares corresponding to chambers of known volume. The white blood cells slowly settle out onto the ruled squares where they can be counted. When the total number of cells on four squares is multiplied by an appropriate dilution factor, the approximate number of white blood cells per cubic millimeter of blood is obtained.

2. Differential smear

The differential smear is used to determine the percentages of various types of leukocytes present in the peripheral blood, as well as the characteristics of the red blood cells. A total of 100 leukocytes, randomly selected, are classified by examining their size, shape, morphological appearance, and staining characteristics under the microscope, and the number of cells in each classification is recorded.

These numbers, expressed as percentages, are designated as the **relative count.** To determine the absolute numbers of the various types of leukocytes per unit volume of blood, these percentages are multiplied by the total WBC. The resulting figures are referred to as the **absolute count.** With leukocytosis, it is not at all uncommon to see the relative percentage of one type of white cell decrease while the absolute numbers of this cell type remain within normal limits.

The circulating leukocytes can be divided into two groups: the granulocytic series and the lymphocytic series. As the names imply, the granulocytes contain granules of varying sizes and compositions in their cytoplasm. Most of these cells are thought to arise in the bone marrow. Neutrophils, basophils, eosinophils, and monocytes may all be classified as granulocytes. The lymphocytic series comprises a single cell type called the lymphocyte. These cells, produced in the lymph nodes throughout the body, do not normally contain granules in their cytoplasm.

The white cells in the vascular system are contained in two pools: the circulating pool and the marginal pool. The marginal pool consists of granulocytic cells which occupy positions along the inner walls of large blood vessels and within the capillaries of the spleen, lung, and bone marrow. Under the influence of corticosteroids or stress, granulocytic cells from the marginal pool enter the circulating blood, producing an immediate leukocytosis. Release of granulocytes from the marginal pool alone can double the total leukocyte count.

If a severe inflammatory process persists longer than 24 to 48 hours, the bone marrow begins to manufacture more granulocytic cells to make up for depletion of the marginal pool. At this time, immature neutrophils appear in the blood, the number depending on the severity and cause of the disease.

Acute bacterial disease and acute stress immediately produce, in the dog, neutrophilia, slight monocytosis, lymphopenia, and eosinopenia. As the disease progresses and the bone marrow is stimulated, a regenerative shift (leukocytosis with increased numbers of immature neutrophils) occurs, while lymphopenia, eosinopenia, and mild monocytosis persist; although the neutrophilia and monocytosis remain for varying periods. Eosinophils reappear in the blood at this time, and lymphocytes increase in numbers. Should the condition progress to the chronic phase, the numbers of circulating lymphocytes and eosinophils may increase further.

Many viral diseases cause leukopenia—presumably because of leukocyte damage and decreased production of leukocytes. This change, which usually occurs approximately 3 to 8 days following the onset of infection, is most pronounced in the lymphocytes; but at times granulocytes are also affected. If the host survives and secondary bacteria invaders are avoided, relatively rapid replenishment of circulating leukocytes takes place.

Although abnormalities in the leukocyte population in a single blood sample can give the surgeon valuable information, serial hemograms should be made in order to follow the progress of disease by monitoring changes in leukocyte activity.

III. Clinical Chemistry

All clinical laboratory determinations can be broken down into two general categories: hematologic and chemical. Although there is some overlapping between the two categories (in hemoglobin

144

determinations, for example), hematology involves primarily the cellular elements of the blood, whereas clinical chemistry is concerned with the concentration of various organic and inorganic compounds in the blood. Since the results of most chemical and some hematologic determinations done on the blood are expressed as concentrations (amount per unit volume), it is important to recognize the effect of dehydration on these results.

The total amount of any constituent present in a solution is equal to the concentration of that constituent (amount per unit volume) times the volume of the solution. A decrease in the fluid volume will increase the concentration of the solution without changing the total amount of solute present. In the vascular system, dehydration caused by protracted vomiting, profuse diarrhea, excessive perspiration, and water deprivation results in a loss of water from the plasma without an appreciable change in the total amount of cellular and chemical components suspended in the plasma. As a result, the concentration of these components is increased, although the total amounts present are not changed. It is important, therefore, that the animal's state of hydration be carefully assessed clinically and by means of hematocrit and hemoglobin determinations. If the animal is found to be dehydrated, the results of the clinical laboratory determinations should be corrected to reflect more accurately the total amount of various constituents present in the blood.

Of all the chemical constituents that exist in the serum, only the serum enzymes are not measured in terms of concentration in a known volume of serum. Since methods for separating and quantitating enzymes are very difficult and often imprecise, a standardized measurement of enzyme activity has been substituted for their chemical separation from the serum. The activity of enzymes is expressed in international units. An international unit of enzyme activity is defined as that amount of activity which will catalyze the transformation of 1 μmole of substrate per minute under defined conditions.

Although the words *activity* and *concentration* are often used synonymously when referring to serum enzymes, *activity* is the correct term; since the amount of enzyme in the serum is never directly measured. In two serum samples containing the same concentration of an enzyme, it is possible for the *activity* of one sample to be twice that of the other. The explanation lies in the presence of enzyme inhibitors and other rate-limiting factors in the serum which alter the enzyme activity.

A. Blood urea nitrogen (BUN)[1]

Urea, the major end product of protein metabolism, is derived principally from the amino groups of amino acids. The BUN is dependent upon the relationship between urea production in the liver (protein ingestion and catabolism) and urea excretion by the kidney. Elevations in the BUN (referred to as azotemia) are most striking in renal disease, where they parallel to some extent the degree of renal impairment.

Because the BUN is affected by variations in protein intake and by variations in urine and plasma volumes (which in turn are dependent upon the state of hydration), the normal range of BUN values is extremely wide (Table IV). Another important nonrenal cause of azotemia is increased protein catabolism due to anorexia. Periods of fasting as short as 24 to 48 hours may increase the BUN concentration. The BUN, then, is dependent upon three factors: (1) the state of hydration; (2) protein intake and catabolism; and (3) the excretion of urea.

Pathologic lesions that may inhibit the excretion of urea by causing a decrease in renal function involve one or more of the following mechanisms: (1) decreased renal blood flow; (2) glomerular injury or destruction; (3) tubular injury or destruction; and (4) increased pressure in glomerular capsular spaces.

Elevations in the BUN are often mistakenly attributed solely to an impairment in renal function. The BUN, although a sensitive indicator of the body's ability to produce and excrete urea nitrogen, should not be used by itself to assess kidney function. Other clinical laboratory methods, such as the creatinine determination and certain renal clearance tests, provide more specific measures of kidney function.

Principle of BUN determination

When serum urea is heated with diacetylmonoxime, a yellow complex results. A spectrophotometer set at 525 nm is used to measure the intensity of the yellow color. From this intensity measurement, the blood urea nitrogen can be calculated on the basis of a concentration curve prepared by using standards containing known amounts of urea.

---

[1] Although the concentration of urea in the serum is what is actually measured, the abbreviation BUN is so familiar that "serum urea nitrogen" is never used.

B. Serum calcium

The serum calcium concentration is not a commonly requested clinical laboratory determination. Alterations of calcium levels in the serum are associated with only a limited number of disease conditions. One such condition is deficiency in parathormone, which can be experimentally studied by surgical excision of the parathyroid glands, one of the surgical procedures described in this text. Other conditions associated with decreased calcium levels in the blood include eclampsia or puerperal tetany, osteomalacia, and acute pancreatitis. Conditions associated with elevated calcium levels include renal osteodystrophy (parathyroid hyperplasia with renal failure), hyperthyroidism, and hypervitaminosis D.

Principle of serum calcium analysis

When a saturated solution of sodium chloranilate is added to serum, calcium is precipitated as calcium chloranilate. After being washed into isopropyl alcohol to remove the excess chloranilic acid, the precipitate is treated with EDTA, which chelates with calcium and releases chloranilic acid—a purple colored compound. The intensity of the purple color of the solution can be measured by a spectrophotometer set at 520 nm. From this measurement, the calcium concentration of the serum can be calculated.

C. Serum chloride

Although chloride is one of the three major anions in the blood and plays an important role in acid–base balance, it is probably the least important of all the serum electrolytes to measure. Its importance revolves primarily about the fact that serum chloride values reflect sodium retention or excretion.

Principle of serum chloride analysis

The chloridometer affords a more accurate and less time-consuming measure of chloride ions in plasma or urine than any other chemical method available. The operation of the chloridometer is based on titration of chloride ions with coulometrically generated silver ions, and detection of the end point ampereometrically.

The silver ions are generated by passing a direct current of constant amperage and voltage between a pair of silver generator electrodes. As long as the current is kept constant, silver ions are released at a constant rate into the solution containing chloride ions, until all the chloride ions have been precipitated as silver chloride. When this point is reached, the concentration of silver ions in the solution begins to increase, causing a rising current to flow between a pair of silver indicator electrodes. An ammeter relay in the indicator circuit monitors the flow of current between these electrodes. At a present rate of flow the relay is actuated, stopping a timer which runs concurrently with the generation of silver ions.

Since the rate of generation of the silver ions is constant, the amount of chloride precipitated is proportional to the elapsed time. From the amount of time required to reach the end point of the titration, the amount of chloride in the sample can be easily determined.

D. Serum creatine phosphokinase (CPK)

Creatine phosphokinase is a cellular enzyme which catalyzes the reversible conversion of phosphocreatine to creatine, liberating high-energy phosphate. CPK is found almost exclusively in the myocardium, skeletal muscle, and brain; only very minute amounts occur in other organs, and none is found in the liver. This peculiar tissue distribution makes elevated serum levels of CPK a relatively specific indicator of myocardial, muscular, or cerebral damage.

Serum CPK levels start to rise approximately 4 to 6 hours after a myocardial infarction, reaching a peak within 24 to 36 hours and returning to normal as early as the third day. The early elevation of serum CPK following myocardial infarction is clearly advantageous in the diagnosis and prognosis of this disease, although the transient nature of the elevation is a distinct disadvantage.

Other clinical laboratory determinations, for example, concentration of the lactic dehydrogenase isoenzymes, are not nearly as sensitive or reliable as the serum CPK. Unlike lactic dehydrogenase isoenzymes, the serum CPK is not affected by the hepatic congestion and associated liver disorders which may accompany cardiac disease. Damage to skeletal muscles (such as occurs in extensive surgical procedures) may, however, lead to elevated levels of CPK.

Principle of serum creatine phosphokinase analysis

The enzyme creatine phosphokinase catalyzes the transfer of a phosphate group from adenosine-5-triphosphate to creatine, forming adenosine-5-diphosphate and creatine phosphate.

In a coupled reaction, pyruvate kinase (PK) catalyzes the transfer of a phosphate group of phosphoenolpyruvate to adenosine-5-diphosphate, forming adenosine-5-triphosphate and pyruvate. The pyruvate reacts with 2, 4,-dinitrophenylhydrazine and sodium hydroxide to form the highly colored pyruvate hydrazone, the absorbance of which is read at 440 nm in a spectrophotometer. The absorbance reading may then be compared with a concentration curve prepared by using standards containing known amounts of pyruvate or creatine phosphokinase.

E. Serum creatinine

Creatinine is an anhydride of creatine formed either by dehydration of creatine or by removal of phosphoric acid from phosphocreatine. Free creatinine appears in the blood and is ultimately excreted in the urine at a remarkably constant rate. Blood levels of creatinine in normal subjects appear to be even more constant than urinary excretion of the compound. Because the serum creatinine is virtually independent of protein metabolism and the rate of urine formation, it is often preferred to the BUN as a screening test for evaluating renal function.

In the presence of renal disease, the creatinine concentration in serum appears to rise more slowly than the BUN; some reports, in fact, indicate that creatinine is seldom elevated above normal limits until less than 25% of functional renal tissue remains. The serum creatinine also falls more slowly than the BUN when hemodialysis is used to treat renal failure; hence, the former test is less useful in assessing the effectiveness of such therapy.

Principle of serum creatinine analysis

Creatinine reacts with picrate in alkaline solutions to form a red complex. The amount formed is proportional to the creatinine concentration and may be measured spectrophotometrically at 520 nm.

F. Blood glucose

The blood glucose concentration—one of the most frequently requested laboratory determinations—is used primarily to assess the absorption and utilization of carbohydrate. The blood, or, more correctly, *serum* glucose level, is influenced by a number of factors, including circulating levels of insulin, catecholamines, corticosteroids, and electrolytes.

The serum glucose determination is often useful in differentiating epileptic convulsions from convulsions due to hypoglycemia associated with a pancreatic neoplasm. It is less useful in evaluating clinical problems in which multiple mechanisms affect the blood levels of glucose.

An example of this type of problem is the glucocorticoid deficiency that follows bilateral adrenalectomy. Of the many hormonally mediated mechanisms that alter blood glucose concentrations, several involve hormones synthesized in the adrenal glands. The glucocorticoids, which are synthesized in the adrenal cortex, not only decrease the peripheral utilization of glucose; they also increase protein catabolism and gluconeogenesis in the liver. Epinephrine, which is synthesized in the adrenal medulla, stimulates the breakdown of liver glycogen into glucose, which is subsequently released into the blood.

The utilization of serum glucose determinations to evaluate the degree of glucocorticoid deficiency following bilateral adrenalectomy is complicated by the concomitant loss of mineralocorticoid secretion, with resultant hyponatremia. Since sodium ions are required for the absorption of glucose and other monosaccharides through the gastrointestinal mucosa, a marked decrease in the serum sodium concentration will lead to hypoglycemia. On the whole, however, serum glucose concentrations are not greatly altered until the adrenal crisis is very pronounced.

Principle of serum glucose analysis

Several methods have been developed for determining the concentration of glucose in serum. The choice of method depends upon the degree of specificity required. Some of the tests are not specific for glucose but will measure a group of compounds which include glucose, aldosaccharides, for example. These methods can be used for serum glucose determinations because the other compounds that they measure are not normally found in blood. More specific methods, such as those involving glucose oxidase, are also used for routine clinical determinations.

One of the methods commonly used in clinical laboratories is the *o*-toluidine reaction for the determination of aldosaccharides. When a primary aromatic amine and glacial acetic acid are added to serum, the aldosaccharides condense to form a blue-green complex which can be measured spectrophotometrically at 590 nm. This reaction is specific for aldosaccharides.

G. Serum lactic dehydrogenase (LDH)

Lactic dehydrogenase is an intracellular enzyme which is released into the blood following cellular damage. It is widely distributed throughout the body, being particularly plentiful in the myocardium, kidney, liver, and skeletal muscle. By catalyzing the reversible conversion of lactic acid to pyruvic acid, lactic dehydrogenase plays an important role in intermediary glucose metabolism. This conversion is an extremely important step in anaerobic glycolysis, since it provides a mechanism to reoxidize NADH to NAD$^+$. Without such a mechanism anaerobic glycolysis would be severely inhibited, since the amount of oxidized NAD$^+$ present in the tissues is very small.

The determination of lactic dehydrogenase activity in the serum has proved to be a useful tool in diagnosing myocardial infarction and assessing myocardial damage. The concentration of lactic dehydrogenase in the blood starts to rise some 12 hours after an infarction, reaches a peak at about 48 hours, and remains elevated for an average of 11 days. This rather persistent elevation of lactic dehydrogenase activity is the major advantage that this method offers in the diagnosis of myocardial infarction. It is particularly valuable if blood samples cannot be obtained until some days after the infarction occurs.

Elevated LDH values are also found in kidney disease, liver disease, disseminated malignancies, and certain hematologic disorders.

Principle of total LDH analysis

The many methods developed to measure the activity of LDH in the serum and other biologic fluids can be grouped into four general categories: (1) determination of the appearance or disappearance of NADH at 340 nm on the spectrophotometer; (2) addition of dinitrophenylhydrazone to the serum to convert pyruvate to its hydrazone, so that it can be measured colorimetrically; (3) addition of methylethylketone to the serum to convert NAD^+ to a fluorescent compound so that it can be measured fluorometrically; (4) addition of phenazine methosulfate to the serum to cause the transfer of an electron from NADH to a tetrazolium salt or to 2,6-dichloroindophenol, so that the colored product can be measured in the spectrophotometer. The last method is probably the most popular, and the tetrazolium salt most commonly used is 2-*p*-iodophenyl-3-nitrophenyl-5-phenyl tetrazolium chloride. This is uncolored in its oxidized form, but when converted to its reduced state, is a highly colored red formazan. Since this colored formazan is formed continuously with the generation of NADH, the rate of conversion of lactate to pyruvate can be visualized and quantitated at 520 nm in a spectrophotometer.

1. *LDH isoenzymes*

The variety of disorders associated with increased LDH activity led to a search for means of improving the diagnostic specificity of the test, especially for myocardial infarction. This objective has been accomplished by electrophoretic separation of the isoenzymes of LDH. Five isoenzymes of LDH, distinguished on the basis of migration speeds, have been recognized. The fastest-migrating enzyme is designated LDH_1; the slowest, LDH_5. The latter is found predominantly in skeletal muscle and in the liver. LDH_1 and LDH_2 are found predominantly in myocardial tissue, and are usually increased in the serum following myocardial infarction.

Principle of LDH isoenzyme analysis

Although the five isoenzymes of lactic dehydrogenase have approximately the same molecular weight, they do not carry the same amount or type of electrical charge. The resultant differences in the charge–mass ratio make it possible to separate these apparently identical molecules by electrophoresis. Once the separation is complete, the isoenzymes can be localized by carrying out the same procedure used for total LDH activity. This can be done directly on the cellulose acetate strip on which the electrophoretic separation is prepared. The relative activity of each isoenzyme is calculated by measuring the resultant colored bands densitometrically. Absolute activity of each isoenzyme may be calculated by multiplying the relative activity (in percent) by the total activity.

2. *Serum α-hydroxybutyrate dehydrogenase*

Since α-hydroxybutyrate is used as a substrate by certain isoenzymes of lactic dehydrogenase it can be used to measure changes in the serum concentration of these isoenzymes by chemical rather than electrophoretic means. Although LDH_3, LDH_4, and LDH_5 all have some small degree of affinity for α-hydroxybutyrate, the α-hydroxybutyrate dehydrogenase activity of serum is largely due to the LDH_1 and LDH_2 present. By comparing the activity of α-hydroxybutyrate dehydrogenase with the total LDH activity, it is often possible to determine whether an elevation in LDH is due to heart disease or to liver disease. Even without reference to LDH values, a significant increase in serum α-hydroxybutyrate dehydrogenase activity is a specific indication of muscle damage—usually due to myocardial infarction.

Principle of α-hydroxybutyrate dehydrogenase analysis

The enzyme α-hydroxybutyrate dehydrogenase catalyzes the conversion of α-hydroxybutyric acid to α-ketobutyric acid in the presence of NADH. During the reaction NADH is oxidized to NAD^+. The α-hydroxybutyrate dehydrogenase activity is determined by measuring the rate of decrease in absorbance at 340 nm in a spectrophotometer. The absorbance of NADH is maximum at 340 nm, whereas the absorbance of NAD^+ and other reactants at this wavelength is insignificant.

H. Serum phosphorus

Phosphorus plays an important role in all phases of organic metabolism. It is required for the formation of high-energy phosphate bonds used in the storage and transfer of energy from oxidative metabolism. Besides being an important component of many organic molecules, including phospholipids, nucleic acids, and nucleotides, phosphorus is also an important electrolyte in the extracellular fluid. Its extracellular concentration is partially related to calcium metabolism which in turn is influenced by parathormone.

Phosphorus is absorbed in the upper portions of the small intestine. Active resorptive processes in the proximal renal tubules, governed to some extent by the serum phosphorus (phosphate) concentration, prevent excessive renal loss of phosphate from the extracellular fluid. By decreasing the renal tubular reabsorption of phosphate, an increase in parathormone causes increased urinary excretion of phosphate, thus, lowering the serum phosphorus level. A decrease in parathormone has the opposite effect. In the absence of the other diseases, monitoring of phosphorus (and calcium) levels in the serum provides a reasonable method for evaluating parathyroid function.

Principle of serum phosphorus analysis

Inorganic phosphorus exists in the serum as the phosphate ion. In the presence of sulfuric acid this ion reacts with ammonium molybdate to form phosphomolybdic acid. The addition of ferrous ammonium sulfate reduces this compound to a blue-colored complex. The concentration of this blue complex (and hence the inorganic phosphorus) can be determined spectrophotometrically at 650 nm.

I. Serum sodium and potassium

Sodium, being the principal electrolyte of the extracellular fluid makes the greatest contribution to its osmolarity. Since the volume of the extracellular fluid is directly dependent upon its osmolarity —and hence upon its sodium content—maintenance of sodium homeostasis is extremely important. Sodium levels in the extracellular fluid are controlled through renal mechanisms—mechanisms entirely dependent upon tubular reabsorption and independent of the glomerular filtration rate. The reabsorption of sodium, and the excretion of potassium through the renal tubules, is increased by aldosterone, one of the adrenal hormones. For this reason, bilateral adrenalectomy leads to hyponatremia, hypochloremia, and hyperkalemia.

Principle of serum sodium and potassium analysis

Although chemical methods are available for determining sodium and potassium concentrations in serum, flame photometry remains the least time-consuming and most accurate means of determining the concentrations of these ions. The flame photometer uses an aerosol of a dilute solution of serum. When this aerosol is introduced into a colorless flame, the sodium and potassium ions emit light—not a continuous spectrum of wavelengths, but rather a mixture of a number of very specific wavelengths. Each mixture, or spectrum, is specific for a particular type of atom or molecule. By measuring photometrically the intensity of light emitted at a wavelength peculiar to the spectrum of a particular ion, the concentration of that ion in the aerosol can be determined.

J. Blood pH, p_{O_2}, and p_{CO_2} analysis

To assess the acid–base balance of the animal, analysis of blood pH, partial oxygen pressures, and partial carbon dioxide pressures are conducted on whole arterial blood. The pH of the blood is held within a rather narrow normal range by several buffering mechanisms involving the lung and kidney. When the blood becomes too alkaline (alkalosis) or too acid (acidosis), these mechanisms readjust it to a more normal value. By measuring the p_{CO2}, p_{O2}, and pH and evaluating the clinical data, the clinician can often determine not only the cause of an abnormal pH but also the compensatory mechanisms that are attempting to correct it.

Before attempting to evaluate the results of blood-gas and pH analysis, the student should review the fundamentals of acid–base chemistry. Excellent reviews of the subject can be found in several texts.

Principle of blood pH, p_{O_2} and p_{CO_2} analysis

Although a seemingly complex instrument, the blood-gas analyzer is really a specialized pH meter. The blood pH is measured directly with a pH electrode; the p_{CO_2} and p_{O_2} measurements are made with electrodes of the same type which are isolated by gas-permeable membranes. The amounts of oxygen or carbon dioxide that diffuse through these membranes into an appropriate buffer are registered as changes in the pH. These pH changes are electronically converted to p_{CO_2} and p_{O_2} measurements.

16

Basic Electrocardiography

C. MAX LANG AND WILLIAM J. WHITE

I. The Electrocardiogram

A. Electrocardiograph

The intrinsic depolarization and repolarization of the cardiac musculature produces radiating electrical fields which are manifest on the surface of the body as minute changes in skin voltage or potential. An electrocardiograph is a machine designed to measure the differences in electric potential between two electrodes located on the skin, and to record these changes on paper. The machine consists of skin electrodes, a high-gain amplifier to amplify the electric charge received by the electrodes, a sensitive galvanometer to measure the differences in voltage between two electrodes, and a recording device for transcribing these differences on paper or some other recording medium.

B. Timing

The paper on which the electrocardiogram is usually recorded is ruled in 1-mm squares. For ease in measuring, each fifth horizontal and vertical line is wider than the preceding four, and the paper is marked at the top with small vertical lines 75 mm apart. Each 1 mm vertical space represents a voltage change of 0.1 mv regardless of paper speed; each horizontal space represents a time interval of 0.04 or 0.02 second, depending upon whether the machine is set at a speed of 25 or 50 mm/second.

The paper speed of 25 mm is that normally used for human electrocardiography. For small animals, such as dogs (whose resting heart rates are much faster than man's), a paper speed of 50 mm is normally used. This speed gives greater separation between adjacent electrical events and makes visualization and measurement of changes easier. The values for the two speeds are shown in the tabulation below.

	Paper speed (mm)	
	25	50
No. large squares/second	5	10
No. large squares/minute	300	600
No. small squares/second	25	50
No. small squares/minute	1500	3000
Duration of large squares	0.2 second	0.1 second
Duration of small squares	0.04 second	0.02 second

To determine the ventricular heart rate, divide the appropriate number given below by the number of squares occurring between two successive R waves.

	Paper speed (mm)	
	25	50
Large squares	300	600
Small squares	1500	3000

C. Origin of ECG complexes

A typical electrocardiogram is shown in Fig. 48. Each deflection is associated with a particular electrical event within the cardiac muscle (see tabulation below):

ECG designation	Electrical event
P wave	Auricular depolarization
P–R interval	Amount of time necessary for auricular depolarization and transmission of the electrical impulse through the atrioventricular node
QRS interval	Amount of time necessary for the depolarization of the ventricles
Q wave	Septal depolarization
R wave	Depolarization of the apical and lateral walls of the ventricles
S wave	Depolarization of the basal portion of the septum and both ventricles
S–T segment	Period of electrical inactivity before repolarization begins
T wave	Repolarization of the ventricles
Q–T interval	Total process of depolarization and repolarization of the ventricles

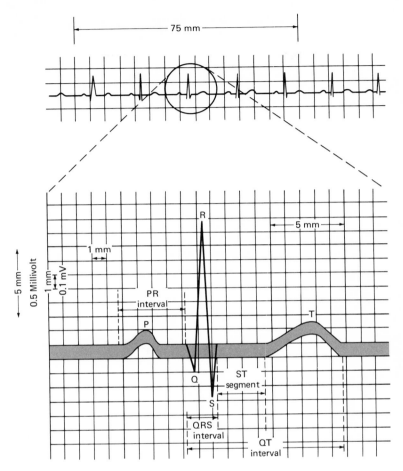

Fig. 48. Normal electrocardiogram. Appearance on the paper and enlargement of a segment showing the measurements to be made.

D. Bipolar and unipolar leads

Two types of leads exist: bipolar and unipolar. The three *bipolar* limb (classical, or Einthoven) leads are referred to as *I, II,* and *III.* Each of these leads has a positive and a negative pole (electrode). The bipolar limb leads measure only the *difference* between potentials recorded at the negative and positive electrodes. They do not measure the individual potentials which compose the force seen as either a positive or a negative tracing on the electrocardiogram.

The three *unipolar* limb leads are: aVR, aVL, and aVF. In order

157

to eliminate all influence of the negative electrode and measure the forces acting on only one electrode (the positive electrode) a unipolar lead system was adopted. This system used the principle that voltage measured at three extremities at any instant will add to 0. The negative pole of the electrocardiograph's galvanometer is connected to all three limb electrodes, thus canceling out the effect of the negative pole on the electrocardiogram. The positive pole of the galvanometer is connected to a single electrode attached to one of the limbs, and it is this electrode that records voltage changes.

If the three axes of the bipolar limb leads are superimposed over the three axes of the unipolar limb leads, a hexaxial reference system is produced (Fig. 49). By using this hexaxial reference system, it is possible to record the direction and magnitude of electrical forces moving in the frontal plane during the cardiac cycle. In order to measure forces traveling in the horizontal plane, six additional unipolar chest leads are commonly used in man. However,

Fig. 49. Hexaxial reference system.

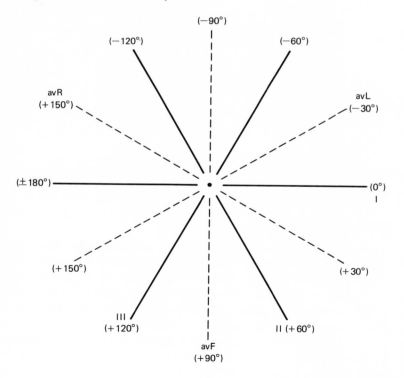

they are not routinely used in animals because of the differences in chest conformation and, as a result, variation in lead location. The designations and locations of these leads are as follows:

V_1 Right border of the septum, fourth interspace
V_2 Left border of the septum, fourth interspace
V_3 Midline, on a line joining V_2 and V_4
V_4 Left midclavicular line at the fifth interspace
V_5 Left anterior axillary line in the same horizontal plane as V_4
V_6 Left midaxillary line in the same horizontal plane as V_4 and V_5

In addition to having magnitude, the difference in electrical potential between the two poles may be either positive or negative, depending upon the direction in which the electrical event is traveling with respect to the electrodes. Forces moving toward the positive electrode will always cause a positive (upward) deflection.

II. Recording and Reading the Electrocardiogram

The primary purpose of the procedures in this chapter is to enable the student to learn how to count, measure, and plot electrocardiographic changes. After receiving instruction on the proper operation of the electrocardiograph, each student should record his own electrocardiogram in order to familiarize himself with the equipment. He should then analyze the electrocardiogram and record his findings on a standard report form such as the one illustrated in Fig. 50.

A. Recording

It may be necessary to anesthetize or heavily sedate animals for electrocardiography, since some of them will not hold still long enough to allow placement of the electrodes and recording of the electrocardiogram. A short-acting barbiturate is recommended for this purpose.

After being anesthetized, the animal should be placed on a nonconductive surface in the dorsal recumbent position. The limb leads should be attached firmly but not too tightly to flat surfaces on the forelegs and the hindlegs. A small amount of electrocardiographic paste should be used on each electrode and skin site to increase conduction.

Proper positioning of the patient and placement of the electrodes are very important in electrocardiography, since changes in either

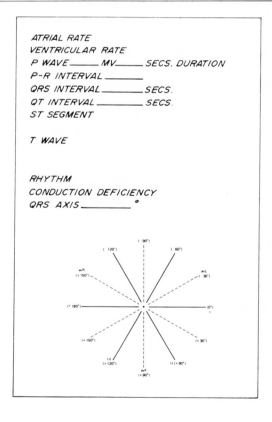

ELECTROCARDIOGRAPHIC REPORT

DATE_____ ANIMAL I.D. # _____ SPECIES_____

SEX____ AGE____ ANESTHESIA: NO____ YES ____, TYPE_____

PAPER SPEED_____mm/SECS.   SENSITIVITY SETTING_____

PHYSICAL CONDITION:

CLINICAL SIGNS:

READ BY_____

ATRIAL RATE
VENTRICULAR RATE
P WAVE_____ MV_____ SECS. DURATION
P-R INTERVAL _____
QRS INTERVAL _____ SECS.
QT INTERVAL _____ SECS.
ST SEGMENT

T WAVE

RHYTHM
CONDUCTION DEFICIENCY
QRS AXIS_____ °

Fig. 50. Report form for recording electrocardiographic findings.

of these two parameters can cause profound changes in the electro-cardiogram.

The tracings from the various leads should be labeled as they are recorded. The length of the recordings should be limited to approximately 225 mm of paper for each lead, since this is adequate for interpretation. After the electrodes are removed, they should be washed with soap and water. A damp cloth is used to clean the machine's switches and cable.

Seventy-five millimeters of the best recording of each lead is cut for the permanent record. These tracings should be read immediately.

B. Measurements

Lead II should be used for the rate, P wave, P–R interval, QRS, and Q–T interval measurements. The *atrial rate* may be determined by measuring the interval between P waves; the *ventricular rate,* by measuring the interval between R waves, and making the computation according to the paper speed. There should be one *P wave* per QRS complex; its height is measured in millimeters (voltage) and its length in seconds. The *P–R interval* is measured from the beginning of the P wave to the beginning of the QRS complex and recorded in seconds. The *QRS* is also recorded in seconds and is measured from the beginning of the Q wave to the end of the S wave. The *Q–T interval* is that time measurement from the beginning of the Q wave to the end of the T wave.

The *S–T segment* should be isoelectric (flat) in all leads. If it rises or falls more than 2 mm from the level of the P–R segment, it should be recorded as elevated or depressed in that lead. The shape of the *T wave* for each lead is designated by the code letters shown in Fig. 51.

The **rhythm** is recorded as normal or irregular, depending on whether the spacing between successive R waves is approximately equal or shows obvious variability. Any obvious conduction deficiencies (indicated by prolonged measurement lengths) should be recorded.

The **axis deviation** is determined by plotting the QRS complex on the hexaxial reference system. For this purpose, the total positive or negative amplitude of each of these waves from leads I and III are recorded on their respective line, and the lines are then extended at right angles (Fig. 52). The point at which they cross is recorded as the **mean electrical axis**. The normal range of the mean electrical axis has not been agreed upon, but it has frequently been defined as varying between $-30°$ and $+110°$.

161

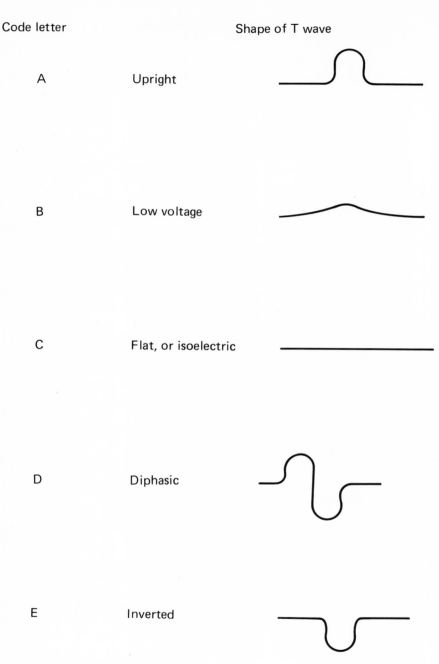

Code letter		Shape of T wave
A	Upright	
B	Low voltage	
C	Flat, or isoelectric	
D	Diphasic	
E	Inverted	

Fig. 51. T wave patterns.

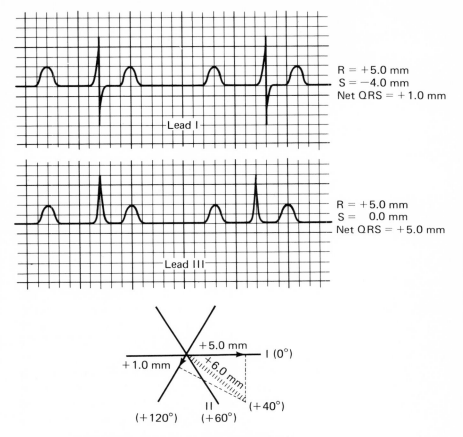

R = +5.0 mm
S = −4.0 mm
Net QRS = +1.0 mm

Lead I

R = +5.0 mm
S = 0.0 mm
Net QRS = +5.0 mm

Lead III

+5.0 mm
+1.0 mm
+6.0 mm
I (0°)
II (+60°)
(+120°)
(+40°)

Fig. 52. Plot of the mean QRS electrical axis.

III. Interpretation

Although the student surgeon should be able to record an electrocardiogram, proficiency in the art of interpreting electrocardiograms takes several years of training and experience. There are only three pieces of firm evidence on which to base a diagnosis: rhythm (count), conduction (measure), and electrical axis (plot). Everything else is an interpretation or a conclusion.

17

Use of the Sphygmomanometer in the Dog

HOWARD C. HUGHES AND C. MAX LANG

Primarily because of differences in size and temperament, the normal blood pressure varies from one breed of dog to another. The *mean* normal blood pressure for all dogs is 140 systolic, 90 diastolic; but accepted values range from 100 to 180 mm Hg for systolic pressure, 60 to 120 for diastolic.

It is important to establish the normal baseline pressure for each dog prior to experimentation. Unfortunately, measurement of the blood pressure with a sphygmomanometer is much more difficult in the dog than it is in man. This greater difficulty is due primarily to the shape of the upper limbs.

For sphygmomanometer readings, the dog should be placed in the lateral recumbent position. The collapsed cuff is wrapped around the upper portion of the top front or hind limb and secured snugly. The head of the stethoscope is placed over the brachial artery (front limb) or femoral artery (hind limb), under the distal portion of the cuff on the medial surface of the limb. The rubber tubing of the cuff is then attached to a rubber bulb and a calibrated manometer.

By rhythmic compression of the bulb, the cuff is slowly inflated until the manometer reaches 200-mm Hg. This amount of pressure should occlude all blood flow through the artery. As the air is slowly released from the cuff, the student listens through the stethoscope for the first pulse sound. The manometer reading at the time of this sound is recorded as the *systolic pressure.* The student continues listening to the pulse as he slowly releases more air.

Diastolic pressure is recorded as the pressure just before the pulse is no longer audible. The difference between the two pressures is called the *pulse pressure.*

Repeated measurements of blood pressure on the same limb within a short period of time will result in abnormally high readings. These are due to reactive hyperemia, which is the result of a decreased blood supply to the lower portion of the limb. To avoid false readings, one should change limbs after two measurements.

When making blood-pressure readings, the student should always be calm and gentle. Anxiety or impatience can be detected by the dog and will cause an increase in his blood pressure.

18

Necropsy of the Dog

EDWIN J. ANDREWS AND C. MAX LANG

The purposes of performing a necropsy on dogs used in experimental surgical exercises are to determine: (1) the immediate cause of death and any contributing causes; (2) the extent of pathologic changes from the surgical procedure; and (3) to enable the student to correlate the clinical data with the gross and microscopic pathological findings.

A complete necropsy (including a histopathologic evaluation) can only be done by a trained veterinary medical pathologist with an awareness of normal, abnormal, terminal, postmortem, and artifactual changes. It is beyond the scope of this text to describe in detail the normal or abnormal appearance of each structure. However, a procedure will be outlined for removing and examining organs, recording data, and selecting and preparing tissues for subsequent histopathologic examination. After this has been completed, a trained pathologist should be consulted to evaluate and interpret the findings.

I. General Considerations

The prosector should be familiar with the clinical and surgical history of the dog. It is essential for him to know what operative procedures have been performed, so that he can give particular attention to the areas involved. A knowledge of the clinical characteristics of the illness, the treatments administered, and the laboratory findings will also enable him to be on the alert for specific lesions.

Should it be necessary to kill the dog for the necropsy, a quick, humane method must be used under veterinary medical supervision. Intravenous injection of a concentrated solution of a fast-acting anesthetic, such as sodium pentobarbital, is the most desirable method. Intracardiac injections should not be given, because leakage of the anesthetic can markedly alter the appearance of the thoracic contents.

Autolysis can occur quite rapidly after death, especially in organs rich in lytic enzymes (the pancreas), organs containing large numbers of bacteria (the gastrointestinal tract), obese animals, and those which were febrile at the time of death. For this reason, the necropsy should be performed as soon as possible after death, before artifactual changes occur in the tissues. If immediate examination is not possible, the carcass should be refrigerated (never frozen) to slow down the rate of autolysis.

A. Equipment

The basic equipment necessary for a necropsy examination are protective clothing, a table, and necropsy instruments.

Although a surgical scrub suit is recommended, a long laboratory coat will suffice. In any case, a thick apron is necessary to protect the prosector from accidental injury and from being soiled with blood or fluids. Properly fitted surgeon's gloves must also be worn for the necropsy.

In addition to a *roll of twine* and a *15-cm ruler,* the following stainless-steel instruments are used in a necropsy examination. The items marked with an asterisk are the bare essentials.

```
*1  autopsy knife, 6-inch blade
 1  knife handle, #3, with #10 disposable blades
*1  pair rat-toothed forceps, 6 inch
*1  pair smooth-tipped serrated forceps, 6 inch
 1  pair iris scissors, straight
*1  pair Mayo scissors, straight
 1  pair Mayo scissors, curved
 1  pair enterotomy scissors
*1  bone saw with blades
 2  pair Kelly clamps, 1 curved, 1 straight
 1  Stryker electric autopsy saw with blades
*1  pair rib shears
 1  pair bone-cutting forceps
```

B. Handling and selection of tissues for histopathologic examination

To reduce artifacts, all tissues should be handled as gently as possible. A block of tissue to be fixed for histopathologic examination should be no more than 0.5 cm in thickness. A sharp scalpel or knife (never scissors) should be used to cut the block, which should contain a representative sample of all layers of the organ being examined (serosa to mucosa, adventitia to intima, etc.). Tissues should be placed in at least 10 times their volume of a 10% solution of neutral buffered formalin. Brains, when saved, should be fixed intact after the lateral ventricles have been cut open.

C. Preparation

Before the necropsy is begun, the necessary instruments should be laid out and the formalin prepared. Reasonable cleanliness during the procedure will aid in the subsequent clean-up. A constant flow of cold water should be available to flush the table and rinse the instruments at frequent intervals.

II. Necropsy Procedure

A. Initial examination

Examine the dog for external lesions, incisions, and general state of nutrition, making note of any abnormalities and their location. Place the animal on his back with his head to your left. Make a midline incision from the mandibular symphysis to the perineum (Fig. 53). In males, go around the prepuce on both sides and dissect it back from the body wall. After dissecting the skin on both sides laterally, lay the front legs to the sides by cutting the pectoral muscles and separating the scapulae from the thoracic wall. To lay the hind legs to the sides, disarticulate the coxofemoral joints and cut the surrounding muscles. Examine all exposed lymph nodes; the penis, prepuce, and testes in males; and the mammary glands in females.

B. Opening of the body cavities

Being careful not to puncture the viscera, make a midline incision through the abdominal wall from the xiphoid cartilage to the pelvis. Next, make a paracostal incision through the abdominal wall from the midline to the vertebrae, just behind the last rib on either side. When the flaps created by these incisions are laid to the sides, the abdominal viscera are exposed.

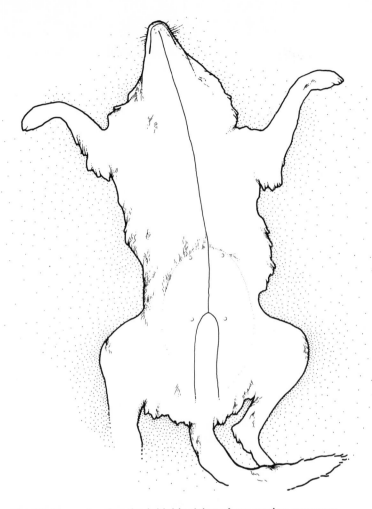

Fig. 53. Lines showing the initial incisions for a canine necropsy.

Puncturing the diaphragm near the sternum, observe the inrush of air caused by the negative intrathoracic pressure. After cutting the diaphragm free from its costal and sternal attachments, use rib shears to sever the ribs on both sides below the costochondral junctions. The sternum can then be lifted off, exposing the thoracic contents.

To remove the pelvic symphysis and expose the pelvic canal, dissect away overlying musculature and cut the pubis and ischium on both sides through the obturator foramina.

With all viscera thus exposed, carefully examine the contents of each cavity for overall anatomic relationships and for the presence of adhesions, gross abnormalities, fluid accumulations, etc. Examine the pericardial sac for fluid before removing the thoracic viscera.

C. Removal and examination of the thoracic Viscera

Sever the attachments of the tongue by cutting along the medial aspects of the right and left mandibles from the rami to the symphysis. Pulling the tongue down between the rami, make an incision across the palate, dissect around the larynx, and disarticulate the hyoid apparatus by severing the cartilaginous middle cornua (Fig. 54).

Maintaining steady traction, free the esophagus, trachea, and associated structures by dissection to the level of the thoracic inlet; then sever the esophagus, aorta, and vena cava at the diaphragm and lift out the thoracic viscera *in toto.*

After laying the organs out approximately in their normal position, make a slit in the pulmonary artery and examine it for emboli. Dissect the heart free from the lungs, being sure to save as much of the aorta as possible. When the thyroids, parathyroids, and associated structures have been examined, open the esophagus and, after examination, dissect it free. Then open the larynx, the trachea, both bronchi, and several bronchioles. Make several cuts through lung lobes at various levels.

D. Dissection of the heart

Two methods for dissection of the heart are described below. The first, which is the more common method, follows the pattern of the circulation. The second, however, is more useful for visualizing hypertrophic changes or infarctions in the myocardium.

(1) After external examination of the heart, lay it on the table with the apex toward you and the right ventricle on your right. With straight scissors, cut into the right ventricle near the apex and adjacent to the septum. Pass one blade of the scissors through the right atrioventricular (tricuspid) valve and cut open the vena cava. In the same manner, pass a blade through the semilunar (pulmonary) valve into the pulmonary artery and cut it open; then examine the opened right side of the heart before continuing. On the opposite side of the septum, cut into the left ventricle; then, by passing a scissors blade through the left atrioventricular (bicuspid) valve, cut open the pulmonary vein. Finally, pass a blade through the aortic valve into the aorta and cut it open. Incise portions of

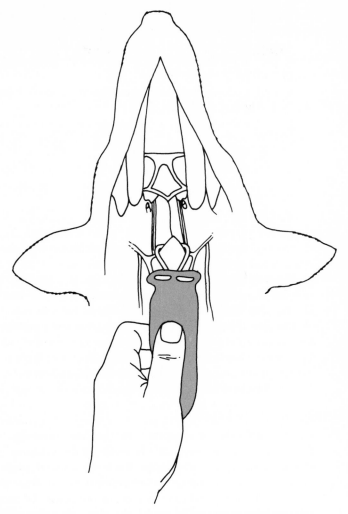

Fig. 54. Removal of the tongue, the larynx, and the esophagus. Arrows show where the hyoid apparatus is severed through the middle cornua.

the septum and ventricular myocardium, taking representative full-thickness blocks for histologic examination.

(2) For visualization of myocardial infarcts, the preferred method is to make a series of horizontal slices, each about 1-cm thick, beginning at the apex and continuing to the base of the papillary muscles. The valves and outflow tracts left in the remain-

ing segment at the base of the heart may then be incised and inspected as outlined in the first procedure.

E. Removal and examination of the abdominal and pelvic viscera and bone marrow

Several preliminary procedures should be carried out before removing the abdominal viscera:

1. Examine the adrenal glands *in situ* and take blocks if desired.
2. Check the patency of the bile duct by squeezing the gallbladder.
3. Examine the pancreas and take blocks for histologic examination.
4. With twine, tie off the cut end of the esophagus, which is still attached to the stomach; then milk feces from the terminal portion of the rectum and tie it off.

Now grasp the cardia of the stomach firmly with forceps held in the left hand, and use gentle traction to lift the stomach out of the abdomen while dissecting it free of its attachments. Free the intestines from the mesenteric plexus and sever the rectum distal to the ligature. Remove the gastrointestinal tract *in toto*.

Remove the omentum and spleen from the gastrointestinal tract and examine them. Then remove the kidneys and slice each one open from the convex surface to the hilus. If desired, the urogenital organs may be removed *in toto*. Incise and inspect the ureters, urinary bladder, and urethra; then, depending on the dog's sex, the prostate or the ovaries, oviducts, uterine horns, and vagina. Free the liver from the diaphragm. Cut open the gallbladder and inspect it. Slice the lobes of the liver and inspect them.

Lay the intestines out on the table after carefully cutting away the mesentery; then examine the mesenteric lymph nodes. Cut open the stomach along the greater curvature, from the cardia to the pylorus. With enterotomy scissors, cut open the entire intestinal tract and inspect it.

For a sample of bone marrow, cut out a wedge of the femur.

F. Removal of the brain

Turning the dog over, make a midline incision from the bridge of the nose to a point posterior to the atlanto-occipital articulation; then cut through this articulation and remove the head. In like manner, free the skin and muscles over the calvarium and lay the flaps to the sides. With the Stryker saw, make a transverse cut across the calvaria just posterior to the supraorbital processes; this cut should extend to just above the zygomatic arches. Now join the transverse incision with a right-angle cut on either side of the calvaria to the level of the foramen magnum. Lift off the calvaria to expose the brain.

After freeing the dura by careful dissection, turn the skull over, sever the cranial nerves, and cut across the olfactory lobes. Once all attachments have been severed, the brain can easily be removed. Free the pituitary gland by cutting the bony sella and surrounding soft tissue; then gently remove it and wrap it in a piece of gauze or a paper towel for fixation.

III. Recording the Necropsy Findings

Unless the findings are properly described and recorded, the value of the gross necropsy examination is lost. The student should attempt to describe in detail any abnormality found during the examination; too much detail is always better than an inadequate description. The most important items to remember in describing a lesion are its location, color, shape, consistency or texture, size, and appearance of the cut surface. It is advisable to record findings during or immediately after the necropsy, while details are still vivid.

IV. Trimming Blocks for Histopathologic Examination

The blocks of tissue taken during necropsy should be examined approximately 24 hours after fixation. If the formalin is discolored and cloudy, it should be changed. At least 3 and preferably 5 days should be allowed for fixation of the blocks before they are trimmed. Whole brains should be fixed for 2 to 4 weeks, depending upon their size.

The purpose of trimming blocks to be examined histopathologically is threefold:

1. To give the histology technician a flat surface to imbed in paraffin.
2. To orient tissue blocks so that subsequent sections will give the desired plane.
3. To ensure that the tissues are the proper size for processing.

Tissue blocks should be trimmed to no more than 0.2 cm in thickness and should have clean-cut edges. All tissues from a single animal should have the same pathology accession number. Blocks are placed in tissue caps with their accession number; they should not be crowded or piled up.

If special orientation of a tissue is desired, the histology technician should be consulted. Processing of special tissues such as the eye, pituitary, brain, and bone should be discussed either with the histology technician or with the pathologist.

Bibliography

Alexander, E. L., Burley, W., Ellison, D., and Vallari, R. (1967). *Care of the Patient in Surgery, Including Techniques.* 4th ed. St. Louis: C. V. Mosby Co.

Annis, J. R., and Allen, A. R. (1967). *An Atlas of Canine Surgery.* Philadelphia: Lea and Febiger.

Archibald, J. (1965). *Canine Surgery.* 1st ed. Santa Barbara, California: American Veterinary Publications, Inc.

Baker, R. D. (1967). *Postmortem Examination. Specific Methods and Procedures.* Philadelphia: W. B. Saunders Co.

Beeson, P. B., and McDermott, W. (1967). *Textbook of Medicine.* 12th ed. Philadelphia: W. B. Saunders Co.

Berry, E. C., and Kohn, L. (1966). *Introduction to Operating Room Technique.* New York: McGraw-Hill Book Co.

Cantarow, A., and Trumper, M. (1962). *Clinical Biochemistry.* 6th ed. Philadelphia: W. B. Saunders Co.

Catcott, E. J. (1968). *Canine Medicine.* 1st ed. Santa Barbara, California: American Veterinary Publications, Inc.

Comroe, J. H., Jr. (1965). *Physiology of the Respiratory Tract.* Chicago: Yearbook Medical Publishers, Inc.

Davenport, H. W. (1967). *The ABC of Acid–Base Chemistry.* 4th ed. Chicago: University of Chicago Press.

Davidsohn, I., and Henry, J. B. (1969). *Todd–Sanford Clinical Diagnosis of Laboratory Methods.* 14th ed. Philadelphia: W. B. Saunders Co.

Dimond, E. G. (1967). *Electrocardiography and Vectorcardiography.* 4th ed. Boston: Little, Brown and Co.

Gage, E. D., and Hoerlein, B. F. (1968). Hemilaminectomy and dorsal laminectomy for relieving compressions of the spinal cord in the dog. *J. Am. Vet. Med. Ass. 152:*351–358.

Goldblatt, H., Lynch, J., Hanzal, R. F., and Summerville, W. W. (1934). Studies on experimental hypertension. I. The production of persistent elevation of systolic blood pressure by means of renal ischemia. *J. Exp. Med.* 59:347–479.

Goodman, L. S., and Gilman, A. (1965). *The Pharmacological Basis of Therapeutics.* 3rd ed. New York: The Macmillan Co.

Ginsberg, F., Brunner, L. S., and Cantlin, V. L. (1966). *A Manual of Operating Room Technology.* Philadelphia: J. B. Lippincott Co.

Guyton, A. C. (1966). *Textbook of Medical Physiology.* 3rd ed. Philadelphia: W. B. Saunders Co.

Henry, R. J. (1968). *Clinical Chemistry: Principles and Techniques.* New York: Harper and Row.

Jones, T. C., and Gleiser, C. A. (1954). *Veterinary Necropsy Procedures.* Philadelphia: J. B. Lippincott Co.

Kaneko, J. J., and Cornelius, C. E. (1971). *Clinical Biochemistry of Domestic Animals.* 2nd ed. New York: Academic Press.

Lawson, D. D. (1968). *Canine Disc Disease. In Current Veterinary Therapy III.* Philadelphia: W. B. Saunders Co.

Leonard, E. P. (1968). *Fundamentals of Small Animal Surgery.* Philadelphia: W. B. Saunders Co.

Lumb, W. V. (1963). *Small Animal Anesthesia.* Philadelphia: Lea and Febiger.

Markowitz, J., Archibald, J., and Downie, H. G. (1964). *Experimental Surgery.* 5th ed. Baltimore: Williams and Wilkins Co.

McGrath, J. T. (1960). *Neurologic Examination of the Dog: with Clinicopathologic Observations.* 2nd ed. Philadelphia: Lea and Febiger.

Menaker, L. (ed.) (1975). *Biologic Basis of Wound Healing.* New York: Harper and Row.

Miller, M. E., Christensen, G. C., and Evans, H. E. (1964). *Anatomy of the Dog.* Philadelphia: W. B. Saunders Co.

Muntwyler, E. (1968). *Water and Electrolyte Metabolism and Acid–Base Balance.* St. Louis: C. V. Mosby Co.

Ross, R. (1969). Wound healing. *Sci. Am.* 220:40–50.

Schalm, D. W. (1967). *Veterinary Hematology.* 2nd ed. Philadelphia: Lea and Febiger.

Sodeman, W. A., and Sodeman, W. A., Jr. (1970). *Pathologic Physiology: Mechanisms of Disease.* 4th ed. Philadelphia: W. B. Saunders Co.

Soma, L. R. (1971). *Textbook of Veterinary Anesthesia.* Baltimore: Williams and Wilkins Co.

Index

179